Hypertension - An Update

Edited by Madhu Khullar

Published in London, United Kingdom

Hypertension - An Update
http://dx.doi.org/10.5772/intechopen.98090
Edited by Madhu Khullar

Contributors
Sona Gahramanova, Berislav Momčilović, Peter Modupi Mphekgwana, Tebogo Maria Mothiba, Nancy Kgatla, Konstantina E. Mitrousi, Nathan E. Manghat, Emma C. Hart, Mark C. K Hamilton, Madhu Khullar, Anupam Mittal, Harmadeep Kaur Randhawa

First published in London, United Kingdom, 2022 by IntechOpen
IntechOpen is the global imprint of INTECHOPEN LIMITED, registered in England and Wales, registration number: 11086078, 5 Princes Gate Court, London, SW7 2QJ, United Kingdom

British Library Cataloguing-in-Publication Data
A catalogue record for this book is available from the British Library

Additional hard and PDF copies can be obtained from orders@intechopen.com

Hypertension - An Update
Edited by Madhu Khullar
p. cm.
Print ISBN 978-1-80355-639-0
Online ISBN 978-1-80355-640-6
eBook (PDF) ISBN 978-1-80355-641-3

Meet the editor

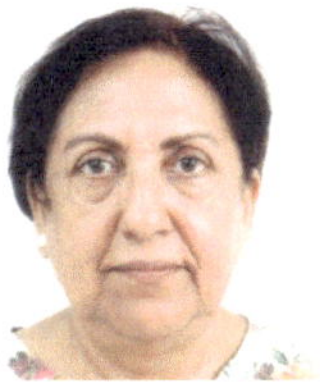

Madhu Khullar, Ph.D., was a Professor in the Department of Experimental Medicine and Biotechnology, Post Graduate Institute of Medical Education and Research, Chandigarh, India from 2005 to 2018. She is currently an Emeritus Scientist, at the Indian Council of Medical Education and Research, India. She completed a fellowship in Hypertension Research from Henry Ford Hospital, Detroit, USA, and was a recipient of the Fogarty Fellowship, NIH, USA. From 1991 to 1993 she published nearly 150 research papers in peer-reviewed journals. She has a keen research interest in Molecular mechanisms, Genetics and Functional Genomics of Cardiovascular diseases, including hypertension.

Contents

Preface

Hypertension has emerged as a major health hazard in both developing and developed countries. It is a major risk factor for cardiovascular, renal, and cerebrovascular diseases and significantly contributes to morbidity and mortality associated with these diseases. Thus, an understanding of its early diagnosis, management, along with mechanisms contributing to its pathophysiology is essential to reduce the morbidities and mortality associated with hypertension.

This book, "Hypertension - An Update", explores diverse aspects of Hypertension. The book has 6 chapters that cover a diverse range of topics, including an introductory chapter on an overview of hypertension; strategies for self-management of hypertension in rural communities; an update on using imaging techniques, including MRI in diagnosis and management of hypertensive patients; using hair and nail samples to evaluate sodium and potassium levels; a role of Vitamin D in the pathophysiology of hypertension and a review of stem cells in hypertension.

This book will provide interesting reading to both clinicians and basic scientists with an interest in hypertension research.

I would like to thank all our authors for taking out their valuable time to contribute chapters to this book. We greatly appreciate your efforts and contribution to making this book feasible. I will also like to thank the entire staff of IntechOpen for managing this book, and for their persistent efforts and expert assistance in managing the flow of manuscripts and materials among the chapter authors, editor, and publisher.

Madhu Khullar
Department of Experimental Medicine and Biotechnology,
PGIMER,
Chandigarh, India

Chapter 1

Introductory Chapter: Hypertension – A Perspective

Madhu Khullar and Anupam Mittal

1. Introduction

High blood pressure or hypertension (HTN) is characterized by persistent raised arterial pressure. According to international guidelines, hypertension has been defined by systolic blood pressure (SBP) equal to or more than 130 mmHg and/or diastolic blood pressure (DBP) of more than 80 mmHg [1]. The definition and categories of HTN are under constant review, and the present consensus is that persistent SBP/DBP readings of 140/90 mmHg should be treated to achieve a target of 130/80 or less.

The ACC/AHA hypertension treatment guidelines have categorized hypertension into different stages: (1) normal (<120 systolic and <80 mm Hg diastolic), (2) elevated (120–129 systolic and <80 mm Hg diastolic), and (3) stage 1 hypertension (130–139 systolic or 80–89 mm Hg diastolic) and stage 2 hypertension (≥140 systolic or ≥90 mm Hg diastolic). It has been suggested that these categories should be confirmed by at least two readings at two different time points, and an average of those readings should be taken. Further, the final classification should be based on the highest SBP/DBP category [2].

2. Epidemiology

HTN is one of the most common chronic diseases and is a major causative factor for cardiovascular, renal, and cerebrovascular diseases and their associated morbidity and mortality. According to a WHO report published in 2021, approximately 1.3 billion adults, between the age of 30 and 79 years suffer from hypertension, with two-third of them being from low- and middle-income countries. Nearly 50% of patients remain undiagnosed, and only one out of five patients have their blood pressure under control. A recent comprehensive report which analyzed global prevalence of hypertension in 184 countries covering 99% of the total world population showed that the incidence of hypertension has doubled in the last 30 years (1990–2019) in adults in the age range of 30–79 years. The prevalence was found to be lowest in Canada and Peru for both men and women, whereas it was lowest in men in some European countries such as Switzerland, Spain, and UK. Several low-income countries, which included Bangladesh, Ethiopia, Solomon, and Eritrea also showed lower incidence of hypertension. High-income countries and emerging high-income countries such as Taiwan, Turkey, South Africa, and Iran showed higher treatment and control of HTN as compared to low-income countries. The highest prevalence of HTN was seen in sub-Saharan Africa, Oceania, and South East Asia [3].

3. Etiology

Based on etiology, hypertension has been categorized into primary hypertension and secondary hypertension. When the primary cause of raised blood pressure cannot be determined, it is called primary or essential hypertension. In secondary hypertension, hypertension is secondary to medical cause such as renovascular hypertension and hypertension secondary to renal and adrenal disorders.

Primary hypertension is a multifactorial complex disease. The causative factors for primary hypertension are considered to be mostly unknown, but we do know several modifiable factors such as high salt intake (in salt-sensitive patients), high-fat diet, high alcohol intake, obesity, sedentary lifestyle, stress, insulin resistance, low potassium, and low calcium contribute to the pathogenesis of essential hypertension. Family history of hypertension is also a significant etiological factor in the pathogenesis of primary hypertension. Several gene loci have been identified which contribute to the pathophysiology and pathogenesis of hypertension. Studies in the last two decades have shown that there is a significant interaction between genetic factors and environmental/modifiable factors in the etiopathogenesis of primary hypertension.

4. Pathogenesis

Increased arterial pressure, which is a hallmark of hypertension, is the result of alterations in cardiac output and total peripheral vascular resistance. Dr. Page was the first one to propose that factors such as blood volume, vascular elasticity, caliber, reactivity, humoral factors, and neural stimulation influence blood pressure regulation. In recent years, additional mechanisms such as oxidative stress, inflammation, and microbiome have been identified to play an important role in HTN pathogenesis.

The kidney is the main effector as well as target organ of HTN. It produces renin, which cleaves angiotensinogen to form angiotensin I, which further is converted to angiotensin II (AngII) by the action of angiotensin-converting enzyme (ACE). This constitutes the renin-angiotensin system (RAS). Renin is produced as an inactive precursor prorenin in specialized juxtaglomerular cells of the kidney and is activated to renin on binding to prorenin receptor (PRR). Renin is secreted from JG cells on sensing reduced perfusion pressure, increased sympathetic activity, or increased availability of sodium chloride to macula densa cells [4].

Kidneys also regulate blood pressure by regulating pressure diuresis and natriuresis. First reported by Gyaton [5], increased blood pressure is now known to cause diuresis and natriuresis, resulting in normalizing the BP. It has been shown that acute rise in BP results in the translocation of sodium transporters, sodium hydrogen exchanger (NHE3), and the sodium-phosphate cotransporter isoform 2 from luminal cell membrane to apical microvilli of proximal tubules which hampers sodium reabsorption. However, chronically raised BP results in relocation of thiazide-sensitive sodium chloride cotransporter also to the apical microvilli and results in increased sodium reabsorption [6]. The kidneys also regulate blood pressure by modulating systemic sympathetic tone via renal afferent nerves. These nerves transmit sympathetic signals to the kidney and increase renin release and sodium reabsorption. Kidneys also are the site of immune activation and have been suggested to induce neoantigen formation in hypertension [6].

5. Role of vasculature

Vasculature perturbations in hypertension include increased AngII, catecholamines, and vasopressin production, and these responses are suggested to be mediated by G-protein signaling pathways. Decreased vasodilatation is an important feature of hypertension, and reduced NO signaling and endothelium-dependent vasodilatation mechanisms are said to contribute to decreased vasodilatation. Increased vascular remodeling involving smooth muscle cell hypertrophy and narrowing of arteriolar lumen also have been implicated in increased vascular resistance. Increased production of AngII, catecholamines, oxidative stress, and inflammation contribute to HTN-mediated vascular remodeling. Vascular remodeling is also known to promote arterial stiffening resulting in end-organ damage [7, 8].

6. Inflammation and immune mechanisms

There is ample evidence that there is increased production of pro-inflammatory cytokines, such as IL-17A, in the kidney and blood vessels in the hypertensive milieu. These cytokines promote fibrosis and modulate pressure natriuresis and sodium handling by kidney cells [9]. The immune activation has been shown to be mediated by increased oxidative stress in antigen-presenting cells and sympathetic outflow [10, 11].

7. Oxidative stress and hypertension

Reactive oxygen species (ROS) such as super oxide anions, hydroxyl radicals, hydrogen peroxide, and free oxygen radicals have been shown to play an important role in the pathophysiology of hypertension. There is an increased ROS production in various tissues such as kidney, heart, and vasculature in the hypertensive milieu. Increased activity of ROS-producing enzymes, NADPH oxidases, and NO synthases has been observed in hypertension [6]. Increased ROS production produces an imbalance between pro-oxidants and oxidants, resulting in oxidative stress in tissues and organs. Oxidative stress can induce vascular remodeling, induce sodium reabsorption in the kidneys, and activate pro-fibrotic metalloproteases [12]. High salt intake and increased AngII production have been shown to induce oxidative stress in vascular cells of kidneys. Both high salt intake and AngII have been found to increase NADPH oxidase levels and decrease SOD expression, leading to increased ROS generation and associated damage to renal cells. Recent studies suggest that mitochondria also have a role in ROS generation in HTN, through inhibiting SOD activity via Sirt3 (sirtuin3) [13].

8. Genetics and hypertension

Familial inheritance of hypertension is well established; however, no single gene has been found to be associated with primary hypertension. Several genes have been identified for highly inheritable monogenic syndromes associated with hypertension, which have helped to elucidate patho-mechanisms leading to high blood pressure. However, primary hypertension has been shown to be associated with the complex interaction of single-nucleotide polymorphisms (SNPs) in multiple genes. Through genome-wide association studies and through gene-specific genetic association studies, more than 1000 SNPs have been reported to be associated with hypertension [14]. These SNPs appear to interact with environmental factors as well as there are gene–gene interactions, resulting in hypertension. Recently, it has been shown that a genetic score based on multiple gene–gene interactions (polygenic risk score) may have a good predictive value [6].

9. Role of salt in hypertension

Dietary salt is an important modulator of blood pressure response in salt-sensitive hypertensives. Several epidemiological studies have confirmed the association of dietary salt with increased risk of HTN and the beneficial effects of salt reduction on reducing blood pressure [15]. In salt-sensitive hypertensives, there is impaired salt excretion by kidneys, and ingestion of high salt leads to increased peripheral vascular resistance due to endothelial dysfunction and increased vasoconstriction. Under low salt conditions, these subjects fail to increase peripheral vascular resistance [16].

The salt-mediated hypertension has been extensively investigated, and it is apparent that besides defective renal excretion, other mechanisms, such as intradermal accumulation and its subsequent effect on immune modulation such as macrophage stimulation, and vascular endothelial growth factor (VEGF) stimulation [17]. Besides this, high salt is known to T cells to generate IL-17A, which is known to promote vascular fibrosis and hypertrophy, endothelial dysfunction, and increased sodium retention in the kidneys. Increased sodium has also been reported to stimulate the secretion of pro-inflammatory cytokines, TGF-α, IL-6, and IL1-β [6].

10. Role of gut microbiome

In the past few years, the microbes harboring the gut have been extensively investigated for their role in several diseases, including hypertension. Under normal conditions, gut bacteria are said to be in symbiosis with its surroundings, meaning co-existing in harmony within gut. However, there is dysbiosis, i.e. imbalance between healthy and pathogenic bacteria in the gut in several diseases, including hypertension. It also shows a reduction in quantum and diversity of the gut microbiome under diseased conditions. Alterations in the gut microbiome has been observed in hypertensive and pre-hypertensive patients and in several models of hypertension, including spontaneously hypertensive rats and Dahl-sensitive rats [18, 19]. Microbes such as *Firmicutes*, *Bacteroidetes, Actinobacteria*, and *Proteobacteria* have been found to be increased in hypertensive gut microbiome composition [20].

Emerging literature suggests that due to gut dysbiosis, there are changes in bacterial metabolites which influence blood pressure regulation [19]. Changes in gut microbial population in hypertension subjects and animal models have been shown to be influenced by a high salt diet, which causes increased levels of pro-inflammatory cytokine, IL-17A [21]. Dietary fiber-enriched foods such as vegetables and fruits and whole grains too have been shown to alter gut microbiome favorably in hypertensives. Dietary fibers are said to increase short-chain fatty acids, which are considered good anti-inflammatory products and also influence other pathways such as renin release by JG cells, vasculature, and autonomic nervous system [22]. Thus, dietary manipulations such as high-fiber diet, prebiotics, and probiotics appear to have therapeutic potential in decreasing the risk and treatment of hypertension.

11. Future perspectives

Despite increased detection and treatment of hypertension compared to the last decade, hypertension still is a significant public health problem responsible for cardiovascular diseases, renal failure, stroke, and retinopathy. This is probably due to several factors such as delayed diagnosis, lack of newer, more effective therapeutics, and accessibility to treatment. Thus, there is a need to develop public health awareness of hypertension, specifically in low-income countries, along with better and more accurate tools to detect hypertension. Further, there is a need to develop newer therapeutics based on recently discovered molecular mechanisms in the pathophysiology of hypertension. Dietary manipulations, lifestyle changes, and immunotherapy will play more role in preventive and therapeutic strategies for hypertension in the near future.

Author details

Madhu Khullar[1]* and Anupam Mittal[2]

1 Department of Experimental Medicine and Biotechnology, PGIMER, Chandigarh, India

2 Department of Translational and Regenerative Medicine, PGIMER, Chandigarh, India

*Address all correspondence to: madhu.khullar@gmail.com

References

[1] Iqbal AM, Jamal SF. Essential hypertension. In: StatPearls [Internet]. Treasure Island (FL): StatPearls Publishing; 2022. [cited 2022 Jul 26]. Available from: http://www.ncbi.nlm.nih.gov/books/NBK539859/

[2] Flack JM, Adekola B. Blood pressure and the new ACC/AHA hypertension guidelines. Trends in Cardiovascular Medicine. 2020;**30**(3):160-164

[3] Zhou B, Carrillo-Larco RM, Danaei G, Riley LM, Paciorek CJ, Stevens GA, et al. Worldwide trends in hypertension prevalence and progress in treatment and control from 1990 to 2019: A pooled analysis of 1201 population-representative studies with 104 million participants. The Lancet. 2021;**398**(10304):957-980

[4] Castrop H, Höcherl K, Kurtz A, Schweda F, Todorov V, Wagner C. Physiology of kidney renin. Physiological Reviews. 2010;**90**(2):607-673

[5] Guyton AC. Renal function curve–a key to understanding the pathogenesis of hypertension. Hypertension Dallas Tex. 1979. 1987;**10**(1):1-6

[6] Harrison DG, Coffman TM, Wilcox CS. Pathophysiology of hypertension: The mosaic theory and beyond. Circulation Research. 2021;**128**(7):847-863

[7] Heagerty AM, Heerkens EH, Izzard AS. Small artery structure and function in hypertension. Journal of Cellular and Molecular Medicine. 2010;**14**(5):1037-1043

[8] Li L, Feng D, Luo Z, Welch WJ, Wilcox CS, Lai EY. Remodeling of afferent arterioles from mice with oxidative stress does not account for increased contractility but does limit excessive wall stress. Hypertension. 2015;**66**(3):550-556

[9] Madhur MS, Lob HE, McCann LA, Iwakura Y, Blinder Y, Guzik TJ, et al. Interleukin 17 promotes angiotensin II-induced hypertension and vascular dysfunction. Hypertension Dallas Tex. 1979. 2010;**55**(2):500-507

[10] Kirabo A, Fontana V, de Faria APC, Loperena R, Galindo CL, Wu J, et al. DC isoketal-modified proteins activate T cells and promote hypertension. The Journal of Clinical Investigation. 2014;**124**(10):4642-4656

[11] Marvar PJ, Thabet SR, Guzik TJ, Lob HE, McCann LA, Weyand C, et al. Central and peripheral mechanisms of T-lymphocyte activation and vascular inflammation produced by angiotensin II-induced hypertension. Circulation Research. 2010;**107**(2):263-270

[12] Carvalho-Galvão A, Guimarães DD, De Brito Alves JL, Braga VA. Central inhibition of tumor necrosis factor alpha reduces hypertension by attenuating oxidative stress in the rostral ventrolateral medulla in renovascular hypertensive rats. Frontiers in Physiology. 2019;**10**:491

[13] Dikalova AE, Itani HA, Nazarewicz RR, McMaster WG, Flynn CR, Uzhachenko R, et al. Sirt3 impairment and SOD2 hyperacetylation in vascular oxidative stress and hypertension. Circulation Research. 2017;**121**(5):564-574

[14] Vaura F, Kauko A, Suvila K, Havulinna AS, Mars N, Salomaa V, et al. Polygenic risk scores predict hypertension

onset and cardiovascular risk. Hypertension Dallas Tex. 1979. 2021;**77**(4):1119-1127

[15] He FJ, MacGregor GA. A comprehensive review on salt and health and current experience of worldwide salt reduction programmes. Journal of Human Hypertension. 2009;**23**(6):363-384

[16] Choi HY, Park HC, Ha SK. Salt sensitivity and hypertension: A paradigm shift from kidney malfunction to vascular endothelial dysfunction. Electrolytes Blood Press E BP. 2015;**13**(1):7-16

[17] Machnik A, Neuhofer W, Jantsch J, Dahlmann A, Tammela T, Machura K, et al. Macrophages regulate salt-dependent volume and blood pressure by a vascular endothelial growth factor-C-dependent buffering mechanism. Nature Medicine. 2009;**15**(5):545-552

[18] Mell B, Jala VR, Mathew AV, Byun J, Waghulde H, Zhang Y, et al. Evidence for a link between gut microbiota and hypertension in the Dahl rat. Physiological Genomics. 2015;**47**(6):187-197

[19] Li J, Zhao F, Wang Y, Chen J, Tao J, Tian G, et al. Gut microbiota dysbiosis contributes to the development of hypertension. Microbiome. 2017;**5**:14

[20] Qin J, Li R, Raes J, Arumugam M, Burgdorf KS, Manichanh C, et al. A human gut microbial gene catalogue established by metagenomic sequencing. Nature. 2010;**464**(7285):59-65

[21] Wilck N, Matus MG, Kearney SM, Olesen SW, Forslund K, Bartolomaeus H, et al. Salt-responsive gut commensal modulates TH17 axis and disease. Nature. 2017;**551**(7682):585-589

[22] Sacks FM, Svetkey LP, Vollmer WM, Appel LJ, Bray GA, Harsha D, et al. Effects on blood pressure of reduced dietary sodium and the dietary approaches to stop hypertension (DASH) diet. DASH-sodium collaborative research group. The New England Journal of Medicine. 2001;**344**(1):3-10

Chapter 2

Stem Cells in Hypertension

Harmandeep Kaur Randhawa, Madhu Khullar and Anupam Mittal

Abstract

Endothelial dysfunction and vascular remodeling are the hallmarks of pulmonary arterial hypertension (PAH). For PAH treatment, there is a rising demand of Stem cell therapy. Interestingly, research reveals that stem/progenitor cells may have an impact in disease progression and therapy in PAH patients. Clinical trials for stem cell therapy in cardiac cell regeneration for heart repair in PAH patients are now underway. The clinical potential of stem/progenitor cell treatment that offers to PAH patients helps in lesion formation which occurs through regaining of vascular cell activities. Majorly the stem cells which are specifically derived from bone marrow such as mesenchymal stem cells (MSCs), endothelial progenitor cells (EPCs) and induced pluripotent cells (iPSCs), adipose-derived stem cells (ADSCs), and cardiac stromal cells (CSCs) are among the subtypes that are proved to play a pivotal role in the repair of the heart. But with only MSCs and EPCs, have shown positive outcomes and act as therapeutically efficient in regaining cure for PAH in clinical trials. This chapter also seeks to explain the potential limitations and challenges with most recent achievements in stem/progenitor cell research in PAH.

Keywords: pulmonary arterial hypertension, mesechymal stem cells and induced pluripotent stem cells

1. Introduction

Stem cells have the potential to regenerate tissues and organ systems owing to their capability of self regeneration and multilineage differentiation [1]. Increased pulmonary artery pressure (PAP) causes right ventricular heart failure, which is one of the main reasons why PAH is thought to be incurable [2]. Two essential cell types in the pulmonary arteries that have been significantly impacted by PAH: endothelial cell loss of function and pulmonary artery smooth muscle cells (PASMCs) expansion [3]. Additionally, the pathologic characteristics that were introduced, such as endovascular diameter constriction into the endothelial cells, excessive proliferation of fibroblast and smooth muscle cells (SMC), and a lack of communication between pericytes, contributed to the dysfunction process [4]. The pathobiology of disease can be characterized in terms of changes in RV vascular capacity, and it is shown that in order to preserve coordination between normal cardiac output and RV ventricular-arterial (VA) coupling, there is a distinct transition from adaptive to maladaptive state [5]. Because contractility and thickness of artery wall are increasing which result in RV dilatation, decreased contractility and cardiac output, and VA uncoupling [6, 7]. Patients who have been diagnosed with long-term RV failure will eventually die. Maladaptive RV remodeling has been associated to decreased angiogenesis, increased metabolic alterations, fibrosis, and disruption of the autonomic nervous system at numerous cellular levels. As a result, PAH is still a fatal disorder with no corrective treatment [8]. Stem cells (SC), on the other hand, are seen as a new cell based therapy approach for those suffering with PAH, as they successfully address symptoms associated to mitochondrial and pulmonary vascular endothelial failure, as well as controlling pulmonary artery expansion in smooth muscle cell [9]. The ultimate goal of SC therapy is to restore cardiopulmonary function while avoiding serious side effects. Another compelling feature is genetic alterations which ultimately boost the effectiveness of stem cells in treating PAH. Adult stem cells are attributed to multipotency with an exception of pluripotent nature found in umbilical cord blood [10]. The right ventricle can be treated using stem cells for instance, MSCs, EPCs, iPSCs, ADSCs, and CPCs. Clinical investigations have shown that the two cell types of differentiating cells which are MSCs and EPCs have been regarded as a putative therapy for PAH as illustrated in **Figure 1** [9, 11]. This pulmonary vascular remodeling process includes endothelial injury and repair, development of smooth muscle cells, and the participation of resident and circulating stem/progenitor cells [10, 12–14]. Stem/progenitor cells have the ability to develop into vascular cell lineages, which may aid in the regeneration process and be effective in the treatment of this condition [15, 16].

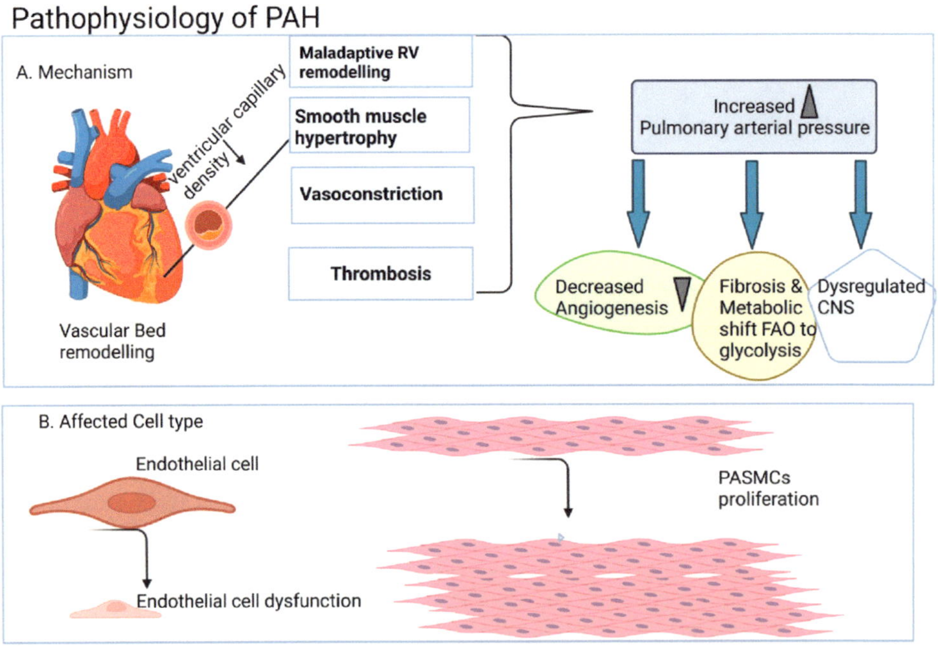

Figure 1.
Mechanism of progression of pulmonary arterial hypertension. (a) defects in right ventricle takes place through decrease in ventricular capillary density. (B) cardiac endothelial cells dysfunction and over proliferation of PASMCs.

2. Regaining of PA endothelial dysfunction by stem cells

The following sections will specifically discuss the different types of stem/progenitor cells involved in PAH.

2.1 Mesenchymal stem cells (MSCs)

MSCs, often referred to as mesenchymal stromal cells, are non-hematopoietic cells that are present in bone marrow stroma. They are a diverse cell population with a built-in capacity for self-regeneration and cell differentiation into a variety of different cell types. MSC-based stem cell treatment has gotten a lot of attention in healing wounded tissue since MSCs are unique in that they can differentiate into multiple cell types and release paracrine substances [17–20]. Such cells can be obtained from different origins such as from bone Marrow, peripheral blood, amniotic fluid, placenta and umbilical cord blood etc. as shown in **Figure 2**. Apparently, the differentiation of stromal cells into adipocytes, osteoblasts and chondroblasts, is due to its remarkable multipotent feature among other cell types. They display specific markers on their

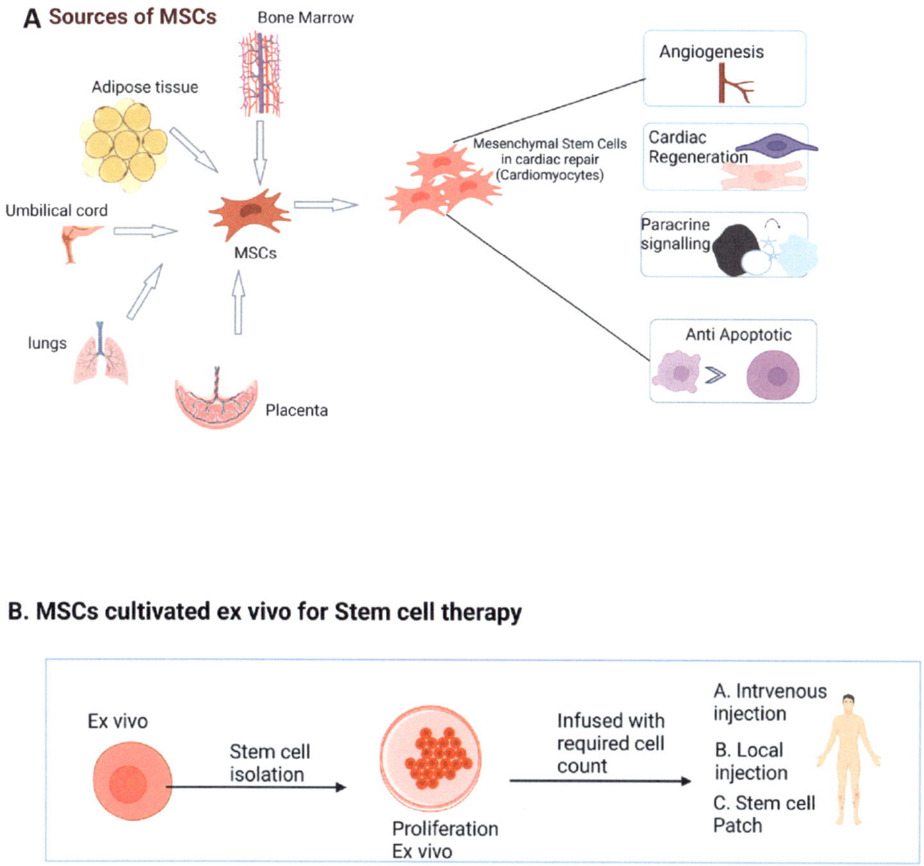

Figure 2.
A. the origin of MSCs and their lineage into cardiomyocytes cells with their characteristics role in regeneration. B MSCs ex vivo preparation for transplantation.

cell specific surface markers: CD90, CD73, and CD105, but not CD14, CD24, CD31, or CD45 [21]. MSCs shows the competence to move to wounded lung tissue and secrete anti-apoptotic (Bcl-2), angiogenic Vascular endothelial growth factor (VEGF), and anti-inflammatory interferon (IFN), Interleukins (IL-10), and Hepatocyte Growth Factor (HGF) proteins. MSC's immunological tolerance is a crucial trait that makes them ideal for clinical usage [22]. In PAH, MSCs are highly suitable for right ventricular (RV) cell therapy because of their tendency to release paracrine chemicals which has proangiogenic and protect cells against harmful agents by secreting various compounds (cytoprotective effects). They may protect cardiomyocytes against hypertrophy and fibrosis by increasing capillary density. Finally, their immunostimulatory attribute make them very appealing for stem cell treatment [23].

As research suggest the Prostacyclin synthase (PCS) gene in MSC's have been demonstrated to reduce right ventricular hypertrophy (RVH) and inhibit monocrotaline induced pulmonary arteriolar remodeling [19, 23]. More significantly, this research found that if PCS-MSCs injected once can potentially improve the life expectancy of PAH induced rats to seven weeks after the injection. When it came to reducing RVH and right ventricular systolic pressure (RVSP) in monocrotaline-induced PAH rat model, MSCs produced from human embryonic stem cells outperformed MSCs derived from adult bone marrow in preclinical studies [24]. Clinical trials done so far are currently centered mainly on increasing pulmonary function, and MSCs have clearly proved their efficacy in treating PAH. MSCs are stable enough to remain at the site of tissue injury and inflammation, and they are also simple to genetically manipulate, isolate, and cultivate ex vivo. The systemic infusion of MSC-conditioned media was shown to reduce lung inflammation and stimulate vascular development in wounded tissue. The release of chemicals that perform tissue healing is most likely the underlying process that promotes vascular growth and heals wounded vascular endothelium. Another effect known as paracrine signaling has been seen, which leads to MSCs engraftment and differentiation into particular lung cell types. Because paracrine signaling is present in modest quantities at wounded tissue, it has a favorable impact on damage responses such as PAH [6, 7, 25].

2.2 Epigenetic alterations of stem cells in treating PAH: role of microRNA (miRNAs) in PAH

miRNAs are non-coding RNAs that are found in the human body and are important regulators in a variety of pathophysiologic processes. Recent research suggests that by influencing gene expression of multiple mRNAs, transfection of stem cells with particular microRNA could alleviate the related inflammatory pathways in PAH [26]. Moreover, miRNA abundance and their activation are tissue specific in both healthy and pathological situations, hence they are of critical importance. To exemplify, some clinical and preclinical studies have already found that the differential expression of number of miRNAs that plays crucial role in prolonged hypoxia condition in the lungs of PAH monocrotaline rat model [26, 27]. DNA methylation, histone acetylation, and microRNA dysregulation all contribute to PAH production. Histone acetylation is important in pulmonary arterial hypertension. MiR-17 promotes the STAT3-BMPR pathway, whereas miR-145 inhibits BMPR activity MiR-30, MiR-22, and let-7f were down regulated in both hypoxic and monocrotaline models, however miR-322 and miR-451 were significantly up regulated throughout the progression of PAH. In PASMCs from people with PAH, miR-204 was consistently down regulated [26, 28]. Absence of regulation of miR-17 in PASMCs has been linked to PAH and is likely to be related to cell proliferation. Overexpressed miR-21 appears to proliferate human PASMCs and their interconnected proteins, such as cyclin D1 and Bcl-xl, in vitro genetic alteration, providing strong evidence for its role in cell proliferation [29].

The survival and widespread mortality of the transplanted MSCs in the injured tissue made MSC its efficacy unacceptably low. Cell differentiation, neovascularization, cell death, and other processes all involve miRNAs. Therefore, epigenetic pathways must be explored when taken into consideration for transplantation therapy for PAH disease, and a detailed analysis of how miRNAs regulation might reverse PAH will be crucial for further study into its pharmacological properties. As a nutshell, another promising strategy for treating PAH is epigenetic alteration of stem cells using miRNAs [29, 30].

2.3 Endothelial progenitor cells (EPCs)

The first changes in PAH takes place through apoptosis of endothelial cells and further loss of endothelium integrity that contributes to pathophysiology, creation of occlusive vascular lesions produced by subsequent uncontrolled expansion in vascular adventitia and smooth muscle media [4, 31]. ESPCs are thought to develop into mature endothelial cells at locations of vascular injury and provide a vital part in regenerating tissues for endothelial function recovery during PAH. CD34 and VEGFR-2 were the first cell surface markers screened out to determine the EPCs, according to Asahara. Currently, cells must display a series of distinct markers to be classified as EPCs, although however there is a closed resemblance with surface markers that are present on circulating endothelial cells (CEC) and hematopoietic stem cells (HSC). The CD34, CD45-, CD133+, KDR+, CD14-, CD146+ are phenotypic markers for EPCs [32, 33]. The limitations of EPCs extracted from adult peripheral blood ranging from 0.002 to 0.01% is that they are in small proportion which is required for stem cell treatment. For accomplishing the required number of cells, culturing of cells in vitro for several weeks is required. It is the long culture period necessary to generate a viable therapeutic dosage. The isolation of EPCs from 0.2 to 1% in umbilical cord blood (UCB) produces far more EPCs in comparison to adult blood with greater number of active cells as well [32]. Despite the fact that EPCs are taken from different individuals of the same species thus allogenic in nature and the underlying capability for immunological refusal must be considered. Additionally, the absence of identification of the kind of EPCs makes it difficult to compare and adapt study findings to clinical practice. EPCs has been shown to be helpful to the right RV in PAH animal models. The study reveals that no direct impact was evaluated on EPCs in heart as whole concern was on improving lung circulation or if they were caused by the transplanting stem cells for improving the pulmonary vascular disease. Therefore, EPCs likely to be potential candidates for treating PAH with RV-targeted cells [16, 23, 32].

The present limitation facing are due to its low frequency in peripheral and cord blood, which is one of the key constraints of EPCs therapy. Firstly its inherent immunogenicity, it can only be delivered autologously. Secondly, the transplanted SPCs have a low survival rate [32]. Henceforth the obstacles to their isolation and identification, as well as concerns with expansion efficiency and immunogenicity, must be overcome before EPCs may be used clinically in the PAH area. Because of their clonal proliferation potential and ability to create blood vessels, EPCs also have vascular reparative effects in PAH, making them a feasible method for pulmonary vascular regeneration [34].

2.4 Induced pluripotent stem cells (iPSCs)

In 2006, Takahashi and Yamanaka discovered that reprogramming somatic cells from human through overexpression of transcription factors (OCT4, SOX2, KLF4, c-MYC, LIN28, and NANOG) has developed iPSc, a novel pathway for different disorders through regenerative therapy as shown in **Figure 3**. Mouse embryonic or adult fibroblast cells have successfully employed to create induced pluripotent stem cells [35].

Human iPSCs share many properties with human ESCs, such as morphological similarities, ability to proliferate and pluripotency markers for their differentiation potential, but their traits related to epigenetics are significantly differ [36]. The production of endothelium cells, cardiomyocytes, or SMCs from human iPSCs can be achieved after reprogramming of human fibroblasts to differentiate into appropriate cell types in PAH disease. Although iPSCs can also be produced patient specific through patient's own fibroblast from skin.

In preclinical settings, the iPSCs derived cardiomyocytes are infused into the right ventricle of PAH animal model and their beneficial effects on RV performance were recorded through pulmonary unit, however although these stem cell therapies still aren't injected directly to the RV in humans. In autologous stem cell therapies, disease-causing mutations can be easily restored using gene editing advances, resulting in the formation of iPSCs originated to produce functional cells which can replace non functional tissues and organs with healthy cells, such as those affected by neurological, cardiovascular, hepatic, and retinal disease [1, 35, 37]. The use of iPSCs in a rat monocrotaline model produced therapeutic outcomes in one investigation [38]. When treated PAH model with iPSCs, there is a reduction in right heart dysfunction, as a result there is a downfall in hemodynamic parameters which are responsible to maintain right ventricular systolic pressure. Furthermore, by limiting inflammation, such therapy has prevented pulmonary arteriole vascular remodeling deterioration and

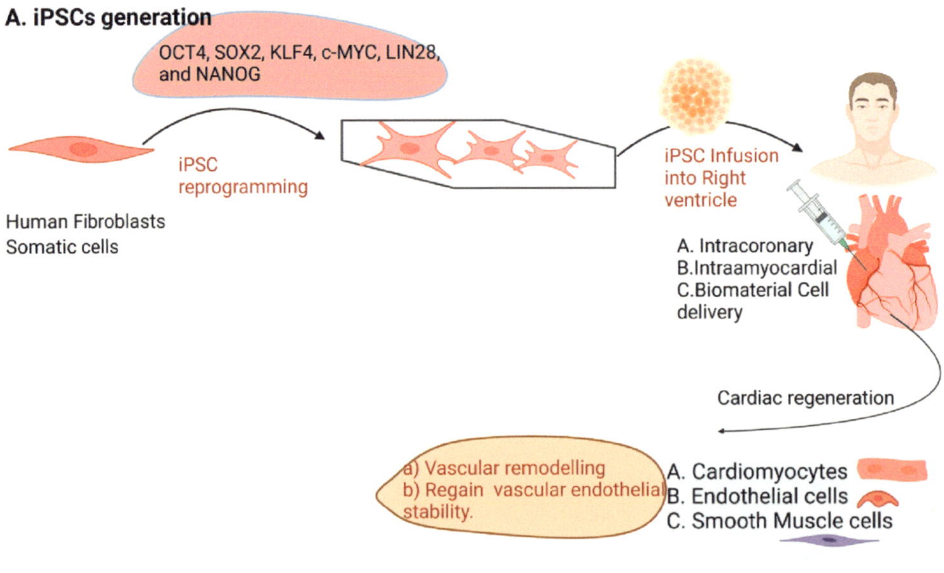

Figure 3.
Development of cell derived iPSCs for cardiac regenerative therapy for treating PAH. The resetting of differentiation of adult fibroblasts with specific factors give rise to generation of iPSCs that can be differentiated into the desired cell type for cardiac regenerative therapy.

reduced media layer proliferation. As nothing more than a nutshell, there that iPSC-based therapy can improve vascular remodeling and making repairs in PAH, as well as restore vascular endothelial stability. The limiting use of iPSCs are due to its tumorigenic nature because of its similarity with embryonic stem cell-like features [38, 39].

2.5 Adipose-derived stem cells (ADSCs)

ADSCs are unique type of adult stem cells for the treatment of cardiovascular disorders that can be easily extracted and grown from adipose tissue. For transplantation, through liposuction technique the ADSCs can be extracted from white adipose tissue [40, 41]. After differentiation, they have a remarkable potential to change into vascular SMCS, endothelial cells and cardiomyocytes [42] for PAH treatment. Most significantly ADSCs are regaining prominence in cardiac research because of its regeneration potential by secreting a number of paracrine substances that promote neovascularization and decrease apoptosis while also preventing fibrosis.

Adipose tissue has a far higher density of stem cells than bone marrow stem cells (5 percent versus 0.01 percent). Miranville et al. [43] used in vitro experiments to identify the subset of ADSCs (CD34+/CD31–) that may differentiate into ECs when cultivated in endothelial growth media supplemented with IGF and VEGF. The cells had a spindle-shaped morphology and strong expression of EC markers like CD31. This group has features that were similar to human umbilical vein endothelial cells.

ADSCs have tissue regenerating potential during injury because it produce angiogenic and anti- growth factors for apoptosis such as colony-stimulating factor (VEGF), transforming growth factor alpha (TGFα), granulocyte–macrophage basic fibroblast growth factor (bFGF), and hepatocyte growth factor (HGF).

ADSCs can induce angiogenesis in models of hind limb ischemia by undergoing differentiation into endothelial cells that integrate into the walls of newly formed arteries and secreting paracrine substances [44, 45]. Research reveals that ADSCs separated from heart adipose tissue propagated better, and possess the strongest cardiac functional recovery, and the highest rate of recruitment to ischemic myocardium in contrast to cells isolated from heart, visceral, and subcutaneous sub scapular adipose tissues.

Overall, ADSC is considered as better option for treating the right ventricle in PAH because of it can give rise to angiogenesis without undergoing apoptosis, and in addition to being autologous, they are numerous, and easily accessible [42, 46].

2.6 Cardiac progenitor cells (CPCs)

The CPCs are the cells which are endogenous and possess capability of a cell for self-regeneration and differentiation that distinguishes CPCs from other cells in the adult heart. They have attributes of c-Kit, Sca-1, and SSEA-1 expression in contrast to others cells subtype. In pre clinical settings the myocardial infarction (MI) was therapeutically treated using CPCs [47]. They're supposed to boost cardiomyocyte and transdifferentiation of vascular cells, along with generation of paracrine chemicals that promote CPCs activity and neovascularization [48]. These features may help the RV in PAH by increasing capillary density and promoting the development of healthy cardiomyocytes. Adult CPCs isolation, on the other hand, is an invasive procedure that involves extracting cells from the patient's cardiac cells. While employing embryo-derived CPCs raises ethical difficulties, autologous iPS cells can alleviate these concerns. Finally, CPCs contain a significant number of various forms of cell with varied surface markers, making it difficult to conclude which will provide most efficient treatment. Additionally CPC, can be considered as an option if another alternative cardiosphere derived cells (CDC) are available, which can be derived from adult human biopsies [23, 48, 49]. The use of cardiosphere derived cells (CDCs) or CPC have potential to inhibit cardiomyocyte fibrosis and apoptosis in stem cell therapies.

2.7 Pericytes in PAH

Pericytes in the lungs play a significant role in PAH. Pericyte multiplication has recently been investigated as an early manifestation of PAH, and clinical specimens with PAH have shown aberrant pericyte covering of the pulmonary vasculature. Pericytes have been found to exhibit MSCs like progenitor capacities in recent investigations, and as a result, they are anticipated to play a variety of roles in PAH-related pathological changes to lung structure and function [50]. Pericytes or MSCs are vascular progenitor cells capable of regenerating a variety of cell types while preserving lineage-allegiance responsive to tissue demands, as seen by their extensive distribution in the vasculature [51]. Pericytes have a significant pathogenic role in the development of PAH because they regulate angiogenesis, inflammation, and have progenitor capacity [52]. For the integrity and preservation of the vessel wall's basement membrane, pericytes and endothelial cells must communicate [53].

Despite its importance in developing new blood vessels, vessels permeability, and contractility, pericytes that just lately been researched in relation to PAH. Pericytes that operate as progenitor cells have recently been discovered, specific tissue-localized pericytes which can grow as the normal MSCs trio of chondrocytes, adipocytes and osteocytes has been confirmed [54]. Pericytes and MSCs from the vasculogenic zone, it has been proposed, may be closely related. Pericytes have been discovered to contain MSCs like progenitor capacities in recent investigations, and are more likely to have a role in PAH-related pathological in modifying structural and functional aspect of liver [53, 55]. A better understanding of the regulatory mechanisms that increase pericyte progenitor proficiency, particularly in the context of cardiac remodeling, could usher in a new era of PAH treatment.

3. Current limitations and challenges of stem cell

Despite the tremendous development in MSCs therapies, there is still a dearth of data on MSCs bio distribution, their target cells' cellular and molecular structures, and the methods used by MSCs to achieve these targets [56]. In addition, even though MSCs are successful in clinical trials but it certainly pose various challenges that must be resolved prior to the use of particular kinds of MSCs in tissue engineering. As a result, improving the bioprocess for producing MSCs from humans and their products will increase stem cell treatments' effectiveness and safety [57]. Additionally, they are important in enhancing the outcome of MSCs-based tissue engineering is increasing the cultural context of MSCs and identifying appropriate target and inducing factors [58]. Due to its low frequency in peripheral and cord blood, one of the key constraints of ESPCs therapy is the long culture period necessary to generate a viable therapeutic dosage. Furthermore, due to its inherent immunogenicity, it can only be delivered autologously. Finally, the transplanted ESPCs have a low survival rate. Firstly, Obstacles in their isolation and identification, as well as concerns with expansion efficiency and immunogenicity, must be overcome before ESPCs may be used clinically in the PAH sector. Secondly, unregulated biodistribution: a significant factor for the limited competence of few cell therapy experiments is poor implantation of rejuvenating stem cells at the site of damage or diseased tissue portion [59, 60]. In numerous clinical trials, the successful incorporation of autologous cells of stem cells in cardiac repair has been injected intravenously or intracoronary in patients. Afterward 24 to 48 hours following transplantation, just a small percentage of transplanted cells (approximately 5%) usually remain at the transplanted area. Almost 99% of the employed cells do not live for even four to six weeks following transplantation [61]. Few undiscovered unfavorable factors in the heart environment or in other organs might inhibits the cell growth, speeds up programmed cells death, and leads to migration to other organs, is thought to be one of the causes of decreased cell viability. The danger of tumorigenicity and immunogenicity is the third and most significant factor to consider [59, 62].

4. Conclusion

Stem cells show remarkably progress in modulating biomolecular pathways, restoring normal mitochondrial function, reversing pulmonary artery remodeling and PAH via improving lung vascular endothelial malfunctioning, lowering cell escalation, and ameliorate other PAH conditions. But on the other hand it is important to note that RV cell therapy should be performed as part of already established treatment targeting the RV and the pulmonary circulation. Patients with PAH who have dysregulation of specific genes may benefit from stem cells modified with therapeutic genes. Autologous stem cells would reduce transplant rejection. Combining stem cell therapy with other types of treatment may be used in some circumstances to provide PAH patients with synergistic therapeutic advantages [63]. Generally, a substantial body of evidence shows that PAH stem cell therapy should be studied further. Because it's hard to know if stem cells are incorporated into the organ and paracrine impact may be the primary route of action of stem cells. miRNAs can also help MSCs with cell differentiation and anti-apoptosis. As exosomes secreted by MSCs can provide microRNAs, it's possible that overexpression of particular miRNAs in MSCs, such as miR-204/206/328, will boost their PAH therapeutic efficiency [64]. To prevent immunological reactions while achieving the same results, exosomes or cell-derived products could be used. One positive outcome till today is that in the preclinical research, through established diseased models, iPSCs have shown practically successful application in regaining viability as curing agents for lung illnesses reflecting stem cell therapy pharmaceutical stability through screening tests [35, 65]. Exosomes clinical trials are now underway or have been completed in over 200 countries, and regenerative medicine requires more research, because of their diverse character, low repeatability, and risk of immunologic responses in recipients, exosomes must have long-term stability before being used as therapeutic agents. The transcriptional and epigenetic similarities between iPSCs and embryonic stem cells are also available as a functional similarity. iPSCs provide an extremely significant resource for determining epigenetic alterations during development.

Abbreviation

bFGf	basic fibroblast growth factor
BMPR2	bone morphogenetic protein receptor type-2
ESPC	endothelial stem/progenitor cell
iPSC	induced pluripotent stem cell
MSC	mesenchymal stem cell
PAH	pulmonary arterial hypertension
TGF-β	transforming growth factor-β
SMCs	smooth muscle cell
CEC	circulating endothelial cells
HSC	hematopoietic stem cells
ADSCs	adipose derived stem cells
CPCs	cardiac progenitor cells
RVH	right ventricular hypertrophy
RVSP	right ventricular systolic pressure
PASMCs	pulmonary artery smooth muscle cells
UCB	umbilical cord blood

Author details

Harmandeep Kaur Randhawa[1], Madhu Khullar[2] and Anupam Mittal[1*]

1 Department of Translational and Regenerative Medicine, PGIMER, India

2 Department of Experimental Medicine and Biotechnology, PGIMER, India

*Address all correspondence to: mittal.anupam@pgimer.edu.in

References

[1] Sun QW, Sun Z. Stem cell therapy for pulmonary arterial hypertension: An update. The Journal of Heart and Lung Transplantation. 2022;**41**(6):692-703. DOI: 10.1016/j.healun.2022.02.020

[2] D'Alonzo GE, Barst RJ, Ayres SM, Bergofsky EH, Brundage BH, Detre KM, et al. Survival in patients with primary pulmonary hypertension: Results from a national prospective registry. Annals of Internal Medicine. 1991;**115**(5):343-349

[3] Gao Y, Chen T, Raj JU. Endothelial and smooth muscle cell interactions in the pathobiology of pulmonary hypertension. American Journal of Respiratory Cell and Molecular Biology. 2016;**54**(4):451-460

[4] Humbert M, Guignabert C, Bonnet S, Dorfmüller P, Klinger JR, Nicolls MR, et al. Pathology and pathobiology of pulmonary hypertension: State of the art and research perspectives. The European Respiratory Journal. 2019;**53**(1): 1801887-1801887

[5] Llucià-Valldeperas A, Frances S, Bogaard HJ. Adaptation and maladaptation of the right ventricle in pulmonary vascular diseases. Clinics in Chest Medicine. 2021;**42**(1):179-194

[6] Umar S, de Visser YP, Steendijk P, Schutte CI, Laghmani EH, Wagenaar GTM, et al. Allogenic stem cell therapy improves right ventricular function by improving lung pathology in rats with pulmonary hypertension. American Journal of Physiology-Heart and Circulatory Physiology. 2009;**297**(5):H1606-H1616

[7] Deng Z, Morse JH, Slager SL, Cuervo N, Moore KJ, Venetos G, et al. Familial primary pulmonary hypertension (gene PPH1) is caused by mutations in the bone morphogenetic protein receptor–II gene. American Journal of Human Genetics. 2000;**67**(3):737-744

[8] Frump AL, Bonnet S, de Jesus Perez VA, Lahm T. Emerging role of angiogenesis in adaptive and maladaptive right ventricular remodeling in pulmonary hypertension. American Journal of Physiology-Lung Cellular and Molecular Physiology. 2018;**314**(3):L443-L460

[9] Crosswhite P, Sun Z. Molecular mechanisms of pulmonary arterial remodeling. Molecular Medicine. 2014;**20**(1):191-201

[10] Terashvili M, Bosnjak ZJ. Stem cell therapies in cardiovascular disease. Journal of Cardiothoracic and Vascular Anesthesia. 2019;**33**(1):209-222

[11] Ding XF, Liang HY, Yuan B, Li LF, Wang T, Kan QC, et al. Efficacy of stem cell therapy for pulmonary arterial hypertension: A systematic review and meta-analysis of preclinical studies. Stem Cell Research & Therapy. 2019;**8**:1-14

[12] Takahashi M, Nakamura T, Toba T, Kajiwara N, Kato H, Shimizu Y. Transplantation of endothelial progenitor cells into the lung to alleviate pulmonary hypertension in dogs. Tissue Engineering. 2004;**10**(5-6):771-779

[13] Kanki-Horimoto S, Horimoto H, Mieno S, Kishida K, Watanabe F, Furuya E, et al. Implantation of mesenchymal stem cells overexpressing endothelial nitric oxide synthase improves right ventricular impairments caused by

pulmonary hypertension. Circulation. 2006;**114**(1_supplement):1-181

[14] Archer S, Rich S. Primary pulmonary hypertension: A vascular biology and translational research "work in progress.". Circulation. 2000;**102**(22):2781-2791

[15] Xie Y, Fan Y, Xu Q. Vascular regeneration by stem/progenitor cells. Arteriosclerosis, Thrombosis, and Vascular Biology. 2016;**36**(5):e33-e40

[16] Zhang L, Xu Q. Stem/progenitor cells in vascular regeneration. Arteriosclerosis, Thrombosis, and Vascular Biology. 2014;**34**(6):1114-1119

[17] Jang AY, Kim BG, Kwon S, Seo J, Kim HK, Chang HJ, et al. Prevalence and clinical features of bone morphogenetic protein receptor type 2 mutation in Korean idiopathic pulmonary arterial hypertension patients: The PILGRIM explorative cohort. PLoS One. 2020;**15**(9):e0238698

[18] Ahn KJ, Jang AY, Park SJ, Chung WJ. 15 years journey of idiopathic pulmonary arterial hypertension with BMPR2 mutation. Clinical Hypertension. 2019;**25**(1):1-4

[19] Yeo Y, Yi ES, Kim JM, Jo EK, Seo S, Kim RI, et al. FGF12 (fibroblast growth factor 12) inhibits vascular smooth muscle cell remodeling in pulmonary arterial hypertension. Hypertension. 2020;**76**(6):1778-1786

[20] Frid MG, Thurman JM, Hansen KC, Maron BA, Stenmark KR. Inflammation, immunity, and vascular remodeling in pulmonary hypertension; evidence for complement involvement? Global Cardiology Science & Practice. 2020;**2020**(1-25):e202001

[21] Nauta AJ, Fibbe WE. Immunomodulatory properties of mesenchymal stromal cells. Blood, The Journal of the American Society of Hematology. 2007;**110**(10):3499-3506

[22] Sharma A, Chakraborty A, Jaganathan BG. Review of the potential of mesenchymal stem cells for the treatment of infectious diseases. World Journal of Stem Cells. 2021;**13**(6):568

[23] Loisel F, Provost B, Haddad F, Guihaire J, Amsallem M, Vrtovec B, et al. Stem cell therapy targeting the right ventricle in pulmonary arterial hypertension: Is it a potential avenue of therapy? Pulmonary Circulation. 2018;**8**(2):2045893218755979

[24] Zuo XR, Wang Q, Cao Q, Yu YZ, Wang H, Bi LQ, et al. Nicorandil prevents right ventricular remodeling by inhibiting apoptosis and lowering pressure overload in rats with pulmonary arterial hypertension. 2012;7:e44485

[25] Behfar A, Crespo-Diaz R, Terzic A, Gersh BJ. Cell therapy for cardiac repair—Lessons from clinical trials. Nature Reviews. Cardiology. 2014;**11**(4):232-246

[26] Parikh VN, Park J, Nikolic I, Channick R, Yu PB, De Marco T, et al. Coordinated modulation of circulating miR-21 in HIV, HIV-associated pulmonary arterial hypertension, and HIV/HCV co-infection. Journal of Acquired Immune Deficiency Syndromes. 2015;**70**(3):236

[27] Xiao T, Xie L, Huang M, Shen J. Differential expression of microRNA in the lungs of rats with pulmonary arterial hypertension. Molecular Medicine Reports. 2017;**15**(2):591-596

[28] Bisserier M, Janostiak R, Lezoualc'h F, Hadri L. Targeting epigenetic mechanisms as an emerging therapeutic strategy in pulmonary

hypertension disease. Vascular Biology. 2020;**2**(1):R17-R34

[29] Sarkar J, Gou D, Turaka P, Viktorova E, Ramchandran R, Raj JU. MicroRNA-21 plays a role in hypoxia-mediated pulmonary artery smooth muscle cell proliferation and migration. Journal of Physiology-Lung Cellular and Molecular Physiology. 2010;**299**(6):L861-L871

[30] Minguell JJ, Erices A. Mesenchymal stem cells and the treatment of cardiac disease. Experimental Biology and Medicine. 2006;**231**(1):39-49

[31] Thiel P, Kaiser M, Ottmann C. Small-molecule stabilization of protein-protein interactions: An underestimated concept in drug discovery? Angewandte Chemie International Edition. 2012;**51**(9):2012-2018

[32] Zhang M, Rehman J, Malik AB. Endothelial progenitor cells and vascular repair. Current Opinion in Hematology. 2014;**21**(3):224

[33] Du F, Zhou J, Gong R, Huang X, Pansuria M, Virtue A, et al. Endothelial progenitor cells in atherosclerosis. Frontiers in Bioscience-A Journal of virtual Library. 2012;**17**:2327

[34] Hill NS, Vardas TF, McLaughlin V. Prostacyclin therapy for pulmonary arterial hypertension. Tex Heart Inst J. 2010;**37**(4):391-399

[35] Singh VK, Kalsan M, Kumar N, Saini A, Chandra R. Induced pluripotent stem cells: Applications in regenerative medicine, disease modeling, and drug discovery. Frontiers in Cell and Development Biology. 2015;**3**:2

[36] Baghbaderani BA, Syama A, Sivapatham R, Pei Y, Mukherjee O, Fellner T, et al. Detailed characterization of human induced pluripotent stem cells manufactured for therapeutic applications. Stem Cell Reviews and Reports. 2016;**12**(4):394-420

[37] Lalit PA, Hei DJ, Raval AN, Kamp TJ. Induced pluripotent stem cells for post–myocardial infarction repair: Remarkable opportunities and challenges. Circulation Research. 2014;**114**(8):1328-1345

[38] Huang WC, Ke MW, Cheng CC, Chiou SH, Wann SR, Shu CW, et al. Therapeutic benefits of induced pluripotent stem cells in monocrotaline-induced pulmonary arterial hypertension. PLoS One. 2016;**11**(2):e0142476

[39] Nishihara K, Shiga T, Nakamura E, Akiyama T, Sasaki T, Suzuki S, et al. Induced pluripotent stem cells reprogrammed with three inhibitors show accelerated differentiation potentials with high levels of 2-cell stage marker expression. Stem Cell Reports. 2019;**12**(2):305-318

[40] Raposio E, Simonacci F, Perrotta RE. Adipose-derived stem cells: Comparison between two methods of isolation for clinical applications. Annals of Medicine and Surgery. 2017;**20**:87-91

[41] Rehman J, Traktuev D, Li J, Merfeld-Clauss S, Temm-Grove CJ, Bovenkerk JE, et al. Secretion of angiogenic and antiapoptotic factors by human adipose stromal cells. Circulation. 2004;**109**(10):1292-1298

[42] Nagata H, Ii M, Kohbayashi E, Hoshiga M, Hanafusa T, Asahi M. Cardiac adipose-derived stem cells exhibit high differentiation potential to cardiovascular cells in C57BL/6 mice. Stem Cells Translational Medicine. 2016;**5**(2):141-151

[43] Forghani A, Koduru SV, Chen C, Leberfinger AN, Ravnic DJ, Hayes DJ.

Differentiation of adipose tissue–derived CD34+/CD31− cells into endothelial cells in vitro. Regenerative Engineering and Translational Medicine. 2020;**6**(1):101-110

[44] Kim EK, Li G, Lee TJ, Hong JP. The effect of human adipose-derived stem cells on healing of ischemic wounds in a diabetic nude mouse model. Plastic and Reconstructive Surgery. 2011;**128**(2):387-394

[45] Cao Y, Sun Z, Liao L, Meng Y, Han Q, Zhao RC. Human adipose tissue-derived stem cells differentiate into endothelial cells in vitro and improve postnatal neovascularization in vivo. Biochemical and Biophysical Research Communications. 2005;**332**(2):370-379

[46] Liu K, Liu R, Cao G, Sun H, Wang X, Wu S. Adipose-derived stromal cell autologous transplantation ameliorates pulmonary arterial hypertension induced by shunt flow in rat models. Stem Cells and Development. 2011;**20**(6):1001-1010

[47] Tian S, Liu Q, Gnatovskiy L, Ma PX, Wang Z. Heart regeneration with embryonic cardiac progenitor cells and cardiac tissue engineering. Journal of Stem Cell and Transplantation Biology. 2015;**1**(1):104-129

[48] Le TYL, Chong JJH. Cardiac progenitor cells for heart repair. Cell Death Discovery. 2016;**2**(1):1-4

[49] Barile L, Lionetti V, Cervio E, Matteucci M, Gherghiceanu M, Popescu LM, et al. Extracellular vesicles from human cardiac progenitor cells inhibit cardiomyocyte apoptosis and improve cardiac function after myocardial infarction. Cardiovascular Research. 2014;**103**(4):530-541

[50] de Mendonca L, Felix NS, Blanco NG, Da Silva JS, Ferreira TP, Abreu SC, et al. Mesenchymal stromal cell therapy reduces lung inflammation and vascular remodeling and improves hemodynamics in experimental pulmonary arterial hypertension. Stem Cell Research & Therapy. 2017;**8**(1):1-15

[51] Ahmed TA, El-Badri N. Pericytes: The role of multipotent stem cells in vascular maintenance and regenerative medicine. Cell Biology and Translational Medicine. 2017;**1**:69-86

[52] Sakao S, Tatsumi K. Vascular remodeling in pulmonary arterial hypertension: Multiple cancer-like pathways and possible treatment modalities. International Journal of Cardiology. 2011;**147**(1):4-12

[53] Bergers G, Song S. The role of pericytes in blood-vessel formation and maintenance. Neuro-Oncology. 2005;**7**(4):452-464

[54] Mills SJ, Cowin AJ, Kaur P. Pericytes, mesenchymal stem cells and the wound healing process. Cell. 2013;**2**(3):621-634

[55] Bisserier M, Pradhan N, Hadri L. Current and emerging therapeutic approaches to pulmonary hypertension. Reviews in Cardiovascular Medicine. 2020;**21**(2):163

[56] Kean TJ, Lin P, Caplan AI, Dennis JE. MSCs: Delivery routes and engraftment, cell-targeting strategies, and immune modulation. Stem Cells International. 2013:13. Article ID: 732742

[57] Petry F, Zitzmann J, Czermak P, Salzig D. Bioprocess development for human mesenchymal stem cell therapy products. In: New Advances on Fermentation Processes. London, UK: IntechOpen; 2020. pp. 203-218

[58] Han Y, Li X, Zhang Y, Han Y, Chang F, Ding J. Mesenchymal stem

cells for regenerative medicine. Cell. 2019;**8**(8):886

[59] Heslop JA, Hammond TG, Santeramo I, Tort Piella A, Hopp I, Zhou J, et al. Concise review: Workshop review: Understanding and assessing the risks of stem cell-based therapies. Stem Cells Translational Medicine. 2015;**4**(4):389-400

[60] Sanganalmath SK, Bolli R. Cell therapy for heart failure: A comprehensive overview of experimental and clinical studies, current challenges, and future directions. Circulation Research. 2013;**113**(6):810-834

[61] Nguyen PK, Neofytou E, Rhee JW, Wu JC. Potential strategies to address the major clinical barriers facing stem cell regenerative therapy for cardiovascular disease: A review. JAMA Cardiology. 2016;**1**(8):953-962

[62] Qiao Y, Agboola OS, Hu X, Wu Y, Lei L. Tumorigenic and immunogenic properties of induced pluripotent stem cells: a promising cancer vaccine. Stem Cell Reviews Reports. 2020;**16**:1049-1061

[63] Li J, Hu S, Cheng K. Engineering better stem cell therapies for treating heart diseases. Annals of Translational Medicine. 2020;**8**(8):569-580

[64] Zhu Z, Fang Z, Hu X, Zhou S. MicroRNAs and mesenchymal stem cells: Hope for pulmonary hypertension. Brazilian Journal of Cardiovascular Surgery. 2015;**30**:380-385

[65] Levy O, Kuai R, Siren EMJ, Bhere D, Milton Y, Nissar N, et al. Shattering barriers toward clinically meaningful MSC therapies. Science Advances. 2020;**6**(30):eaba6884

Chapter 3

Perspective Chapter: Hypertension with a Focus on Comprehensive Magnetic Resonance Imaging

Konstantina E. Mitrousi, Emma C. Hart, Mark C.K. Hamilton and Nathan E. Manghat

Abstract

Arterial hypertension is a leading cause of mortality, affecting at least a quarter of the adult population, with its effects having devastating consequences to the global economy. Unfortunately, the underlying causes and pathophysiology of the disease often remain unclear. Ongoing research in this important field investigates the mechanisms involved in the genesis of hypertension. Magnetic resonance imaging is a well-established imaging technique that is widely used for anatomical organ and vascular evaluation. According to the latest European Society of Hypertension (ESC) guidelines, cardiovascular magnetic resonance can be used in the assessment of hypertensive patients. But the authors advocate a more comprehensive and multisystem use of the varied and novel sequences of MRI scanners to provide an even better understanding of the development of hypertension and its consequences. The extensive and detailed data that can be derived, with the additive focus on the concept of the 'selfish brain hypothesis', might further assist us in altering and providing a more individualised therapeutic approach to one of the greatest non-communicable causes of human mortality and morbidity.

Keywords: hypertension, cardiac magnetic resonance, electrocardiogram, aortic disease, pathophysiology

1. Introduction

Hypertension has been identified as a disease for more than 150 years [1] and is a major contributor to mortality affecting at least a quarter of the adult population [2] with devastating financial effects on national healthcare systems worldwide [3].

Several risk factors for the development of persistently elevated BP, including genetic variations, age, obesity, insulin resistance, high alcohol consumption, increased sodium intake and stress, have been identified and are well established. Unfortunately, despite the leading role of hypertension in global mortality, the detrimental effects, and the enormous economic burden it carries [3–5], the primary causes and predictive factors for the development of hypertension in >90% of patients remain elusive [4–6].

IntechOpen

This could explain the fact that, despite various antihypertensive medications, there is poor blood pressure (BP) control in >50% of hypertensive patients [7].

Given that essential hypertension is one of the major modifiable cardiovascular risk factors, understanding the pathophysiology and uncovering its possible root causative mechanism(s) would have a tremendous public health impact. This, of course, could lead to more efficient and bespoke antihypertensive treatments, including prediction or even the prevention of the development of the disease and its detrimental consequences altogether.

Furthermore, according to recent statistics from the 2014 Health survey for England, hypertension is refractory to treatment in ≤20–30% of cases despite the availability of numerous classes of antihypertensives, and finding a primary cause could improve treatment of such refractory hypertension.

As per Hypertension European Society of Cardiology (ESC) guidelines, patients should be thoroughly screened for potentially treatable secondary causes, such as aortic coarctation, adrenal adenomas, phaeochromocytoma, renal artery stenosis, occult chronic renal disease, and evidence of hypertension-mediated organ damage (HMOD) [8].

This chapter has a focus on the use of magnetic resonance imaging (MRI) which can be introduced, currently in appropriately selected individuals, as a safe and effective screening modality for secondary hypertension and end-organ damage evaluation without the use of ionising radiation imaging [9].

Cardiac MRI (CMR) is the gold standard non-invasive imaging technique for the assessment of cardiac anatomy and function [10], but MRI is also well established in cerebral and cerebrovascular imaging, aortic and abdominal visceral assessment. Aside from anatomical delineation, there are numerous sequences that are regularly employed for detailed tissue characterisation, tissue mapping, myocardial strain imaging, myocardial replacement fibrosis and infarction evaluation, contrast and non-contrast angiography, and phase contrast vessel flow imaging [11–13].

By combining these sequences, comprehensive imaging protocols can be established and the patient investigated in a single hospital episode; this may, therefore, alleviate the need for and higher cost of other multiple investigations, for example, echocardiography, abdominal/renal ultrasound, carotid and vertebral duplex sonography, computed tomography (CT) angiography, etc. [9].

MRI is not touted as a substitute for a detailed history, physical examination, and the usual necessary metabolic/biochemical investigations e.g. endocrine tumours may not always be in typical location.

2. Hypertension and cardiovascular magnetic resonance imaging

2.1 Hypertension and the 'selfish brain hypothesis'

There is a well-documented relationship between increased sympathetic nerve activity and hypertension but the primary cause is still to be established [14]. Early on, one of the proposed pathologic hypotheses has been that an increase in BP is an essential response to thickened and narrowed blood vessels to provide more blood supply to organs. This line of pathologic investigation has been mired in the classic difficulty of determining if the arterial luminal narrowing is the cause or effect of hypertension.

The effect of hypertension on the cerebrovascular structure is often described through the pathophysiology of vessel remodelling and decrease in luminal diameter leading to decreased blood flow [15–17]. But is it possible that the reverse hypothesis could be true whereby cerebral vessel remodelling precedes and is even a cause of hypertension? The answer to this, we believe, is 'yes'.

The archaic term 'vasomotor center', currently known as the rostral ventrolateral medulla, is the area involved with the basal sympathetic activity and supplied by the vertebral artery; disruption of vertebral artery flow may increase systemic BP.

At the beginning of the twentieth century using canine models, Harvey Cushing indicated that reduced cerebral blood flow due to increased intracranial pressure led to increased blood pressure [17]. Later, animal and post-mortem human studies by Cates and Dickinson proposed that narrow vertebral arteries lead to brain stem hypoperfusion and subsequently to a vital increase of blood pressure as a protective mechanism to maintain cerebral blood flow to the brain stem in the case of stenotic vertebral arteries; this theory is known as Cushing's mechanism or the 'selfish brain hypothesis' of hypertension. This mechanism triggers sympathetic overdrive and hypertension to maintain brain stem perfusion [15, 16].

Using magnetic resonance (MR) angiography and MR phase-contrast imaging, our group has been investigating the association of the 'selfish brain hypothesis' with high BP in conscious adults. The data has shown, for the first time, that congenital variants in the cerebral circulation may be the trigger for hypertension rather than the result [18].

3-dimensional MR angiography can help to illustrate the cerebral anatomy of the circle of Willis and the vertebral arteries. **Figure 1** shows normal anatomy.

The higher prevalence of cerebrovascular variants whereby vertebral artery hypoplasia/absence (VAH) and incomplete posterior circle of Willis (ipCoW) is strongly associated with increased cerebrovascular resistance and reduced cerebral blood flow in hypertensive patients in comparison to healthy adults [18]. We have also shown this in a large cohort of young-onset hypertensive patients [19] with a possible link between the 'selfish brain' hypothesis (**Figure 2**). Cerebral blood flow can also be measured at mid-neck level prior to the common carotid artery bifurcation; in

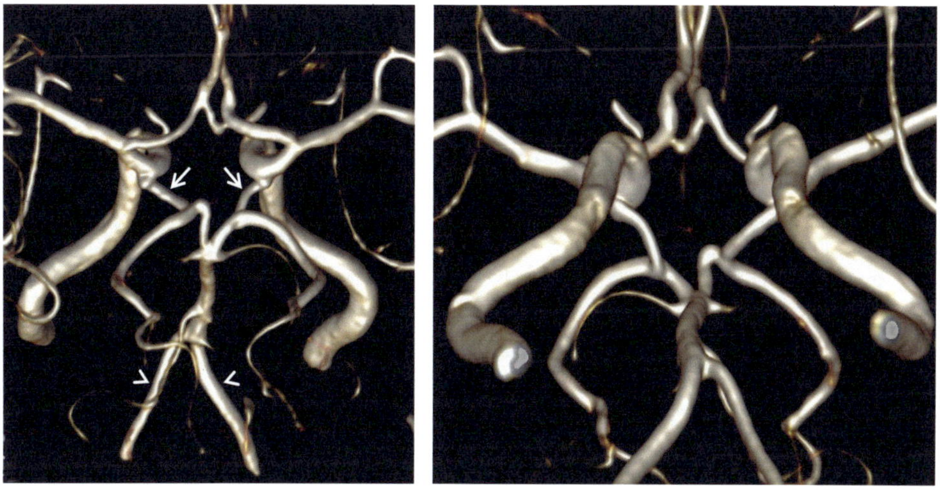

(a) (b)

Figure 1.
Normal anatomy. (a) – superior view and (b) – inferior view, showing an intact circle of Willis with normal-sized posterior communicating arteries (white arrows) and normal-sized vertebral arteries (white arrowheads).

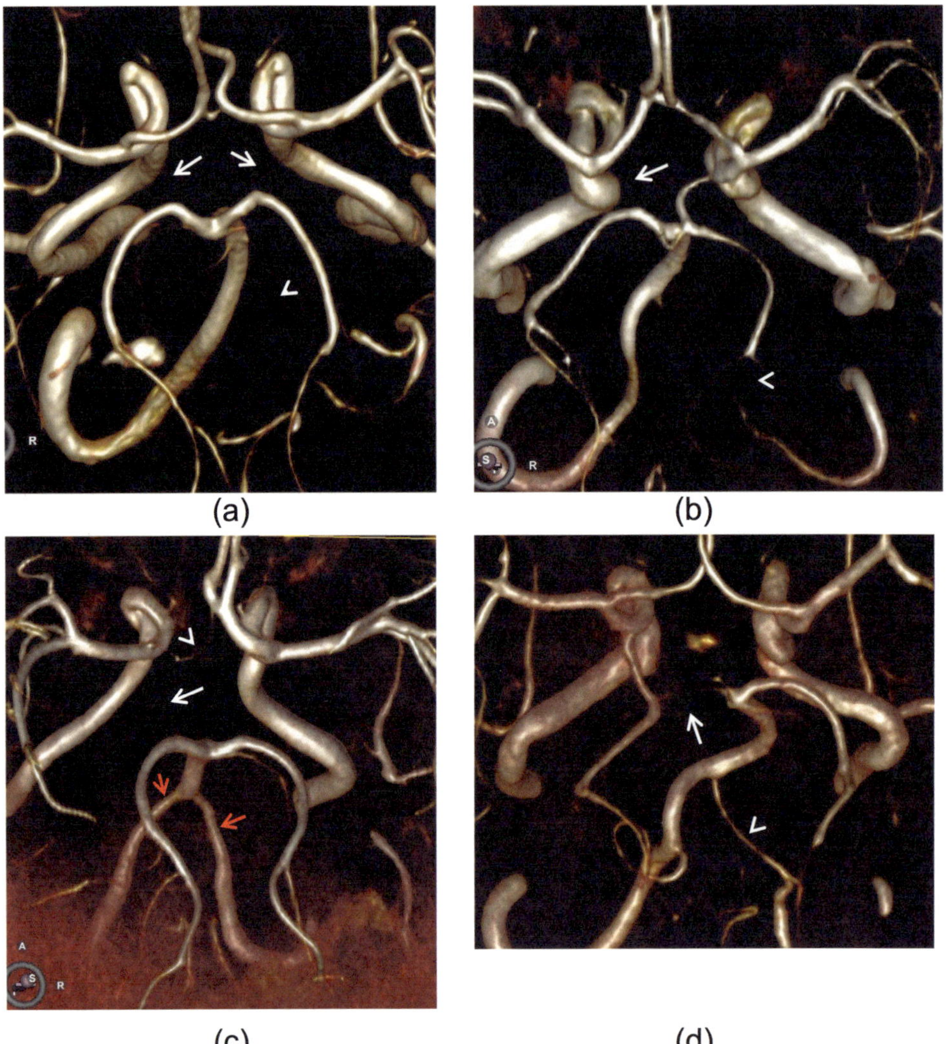

Figure 2.
Variant circle of Willis anatomy found in patients with young-onset hypertension. Superior projection 3-dimensional MRI angiography. (a) – Bilateral absent posterior communicating arteries (white arrows) and absent right vertebral artery (white arrowhead). (b) – Absent left posterior communicating artery (white arrow) and severely hypoplastic, interrupted right vertebral artery (white arrowhead); left vertebral artery stenosis in the V4 segment is also noted. (c) – Absent left posterior communicating artery (white arrow), bilateral small calibre distal vertebral arteries just prior to the basilar arterial confluence (red arrows); note also the severely hypoplastic left A1 segment of the left anterior cerebral artery (white arrowhead). (d) – Foetal-type left posterior cerebral artery (PCA) with absent left P1 segment of the PCA (white arrow), and a hypoplastic right vertebral artery (white arrowhead).

the presence of upstream anomalies of the posterior circulation, the split percentage vertebral arterial flows are significantly reduced.

We have found similar results in a cohort of persistently hypertensive patients post-coarctation repair which could guide subsequent treatment [20]. According to this study, cerebrovascular variants of the posterior circulation as manifested by VAH + ipCoW are more common in patients with repaired coarctation (CoA) and are independent predictors of hypertension or difficult to treat hypertension post-CoA repair in contrast with age and specific type of repair. This may, of course, affect interventional treatment strategy in the form of aortic arch stenting and whether to cover the subclavian artery or a variant arch origin of the vertebral artery in the context of upstream variants that might predispose to or cause hypertension; thus, an intervention intended to treat hypertension may in fact exacerbate the problem unless an appropriate alternative or hybrid arch vessel revascularization strategy is employed.

This is a strong indication that the increase in cerebrovascular resistance caused by congenital cerebrovascular variants is actually the trigger for the increase in sympathetic nerve activity and hypertension. This finding is in accordance with the theory proposed by Dickinson back in 1959. Additionally, this study interestingly showed that cerebral blood flow was normal in hypertensive patients without treatment but diminished in those on treatment with controlled blood pressure. This observation may have important implications in the treatment strategy for hypertensive patients and may change the diagnostic and therapeutic approach; indeed, some patients rendered 'normotensive' may present with soft occult neurological signs of poor concentration, impaired memory, or 'brain fog'. Further longitudinal studies are needed to confirm these results.

2.2 Hypertension and the electrocardiogram

Left ventricular hypertrophy (LVH) is a common finding in hypertensive patients due to the increased workload of the left ventricle [21]. The presence of LVH in hypertensive patients is known to have significant implications in prognosis and treatment strategies [22–25]. The 12-lead electrocardiogram (ECG) is widely used to detect LVH [8] and it is well validated against echocardiography [26].

As per European Society of Cardiology (ESC) guidelines, a 12-lead ECG is required for the assessment of hypertensive patients and specific ECG criteria for left ventricular hypertrophy are well established [8] and validated against echocardiography [26].

The diagnostic performance of the above criteria against CMR, the gold standard, non-invasive technique for the assessment of left ventricular mass (LVM) can be evaluated.

It is also well documented that hypertension frequently coexists with obesity [27]. Due to discrepancy between previous echocardiography studies about the effect of obesity on the ECG capacity of detecting LVH, the ECG criteria for LVH can be recalibrated against CMR measurements by using the steady-state free precession sequence. This study also went through the impact of obesity, over the diagnostic performance of ECG in detecting LVH, thus creating new novel obesity-specific partition values to increase the diagnostic accuracy of ECG in this specific patient's category [28].

In hypertensive patients, the left ventricular ECG strain pattern (≥1 mm concave downsloping ST-segment depression and T-wave inversion in the lateral leads) [29] is associated with increased cardiovascular risk in hypertensive individuals [30] with the underlying mechanisms being unclear.

A great advantage of CMR is its unique ability for advanced myocardial tissue characterisation [11].

Myocardial fibrosis is an established histologic element of hypertensive heart disease; the presence is known to adversely affect prognosis [31]. Left ventricular systolic dysfunction in hypertension, characterised by myocardial strain impairment, has been documented in previous CMR studies [32].

Taking the above facts into consideration using these CMR techniques, a strong association between ECG strain pattern, increased interstitial fibrosis and myocardial systolic dysfunction [33] can be demonstrated; the ECG strain pattern in hypertensive patients is linked to significant LVH and interstitial fibrosis. There is also an association between ECG strain and significant impairment of circumferential strain, even with preserved left ventricular ejection fraction (LVEF) [34].

Obesity is also strongly associated with a left atrial enlargement (LAE), an index of diastolic dysfunction [35], and also a common finding in hypertensive patients, identifiable on ECG [36]. LAE is an index of diastolic dysfunction [35] with important prognostic and therapeutic implications; [37] the ECG may demonstrate LAE [36]. The diagnostic performance of the ECG in identifying LAE has also already been validated against echocardiography [38].

The diagnostic accuracy of ECG criteria of LAE against the CMR gold standard and the possible effect of obesity was explored; [39] all the ECG criteria are more specific than sensitive at identifying LAE and less specific when obesity is present. According to these findings, clinicians should not rely solely on ECG for the exclusion of LAE, and always take into consideration the patient's body mass index (BMI).

2.3 Hypertension and left ventricular hypertrophy

Systolic hypertension increases the LV afterload because the LV must work harder to eject blood into the aorta; the aortic valve will not open until the pressure generated in the left ventricle is higher than the elevated blood pressure in the aorta. In the presence of chronic afterload increase, the LV receives constant mechanical stress which results in hypertrophy [20].

Different phenotypes of hypertensive heart disease (HHD) are well-documented [40]. Even though asymmetric patterns of LVH have been previously investigated with 2-dimensional echocardiography, [41] CMR has shown the prevalence of asymmetric hypertrophic patterns in hypertension [42], a pattern previously described with aortic stenosis [43].

There is an increasingly well-recognised spectrum of hypertrophic LV patterns in hypertensive heart disease with variable cardiovascular prognosis and unknown pathophysiology [40]. Using multiparametric CMR, the significant differences between these phenotypes may explain the varying cardiovascular prognosis and change the therapeutic process [44].

There are three well-defined LV phenotypes—normal structure (normal LV mass and relative wall thickness), concentric remodelling (normal LV mass with increased relative wall thickness and elevated mass/volume ratio), and LVH (symmetric, asymmetric, and eccentric) [40]. Eccentric and concentric LVH is linked to significant intracellular and interstitial expansion and strain impairment. This could explain the varying cardiovascular prognosis following each hypertensive left ventricular phenotype and have an impact on hypertension treatment (**Figure 3**) [44].

The presence of LVH in hypertensive individuals can have a differential diagnosis of hypertensive heart disease (HHD) and hypertrophic cardiomyopathy (HCM); it can be difficult to distinguish between them. Novel predictors of HHD over HCM have been identified [45].

Hypertrophic cardiomyopathy (HCM) is defined by left ventricular end-diastolic thickness ≥ 15 mm, not solely explained by abnormal loading conditions [46]. As asymmetric LV phenotype is commonly seen in both HHD and HCM, it may be difficult to distinguish between the two pathologies; it is acknowledged that HCM and HHD can, of course, co-exist. The investigation has indicated that an acute aortoseptal angulation (angle between a line drawn along the RV side of the interventricular septum and

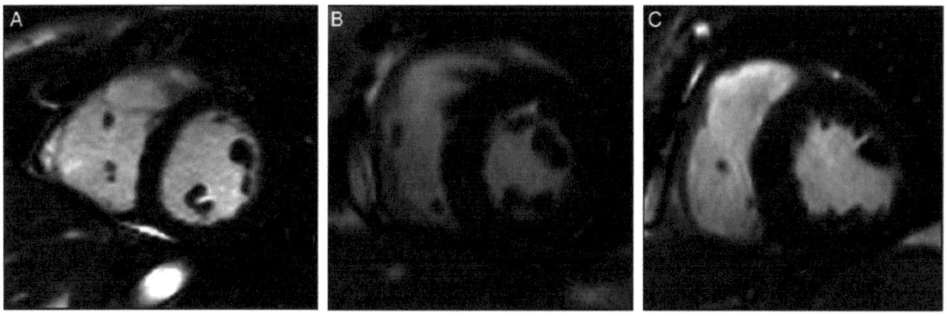

Figure 3.
Forms of hypertensive heart disease. (A) – Normal, (B) – concentric LV hypertrophy, and (C) – asymmetric LV hypertrophy.

a line drawn through the long axis of the aortic root; reflecting a reduced angle from ~130 degrees to 90 degrees or less) and reduced aortic distensibility advocate over HHD [45]. This reduction in aortoseptal angulation is interesting in that the altered LV outflow tract geometry may cause a greater effect on the basal interventricular septum in a region of increased wall stress during ventricular systole, thus contributing to the consequent asymmetric hypertrophy (**Figure 4**).

The reduction in the aortoseptal angle is a complex phenomenon; it likely occurs in part secondary to ageing, hypertensive, and/or atherosclerotic thoracic aortic/

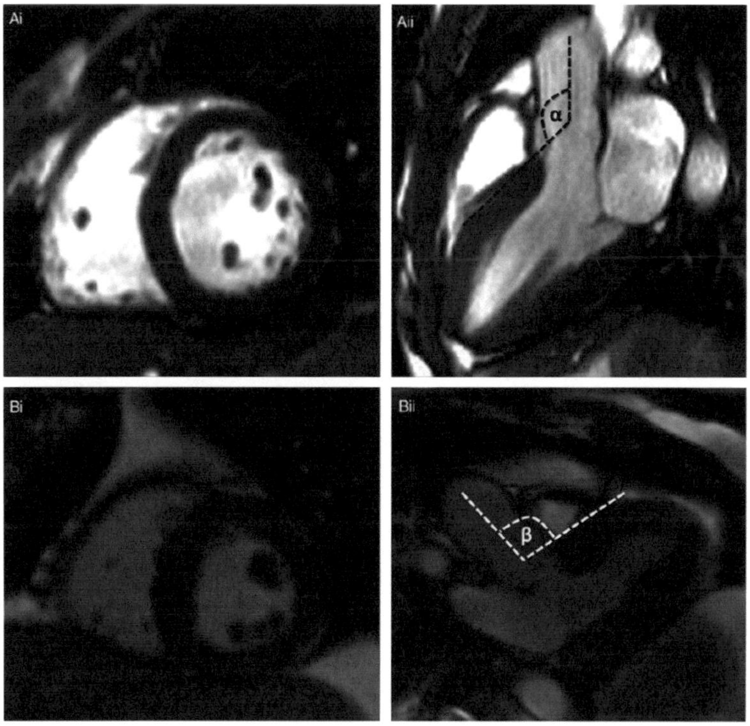

Figure 4.
Aortoseptal angulation. Aortoseptal angle is measured from the 3-chamber steady-state free precession cine at end-systole. Ai – hypertensive patient with no LV asymmetry, Aii – aortoseptal angle = 123 degrees. Bi = hypertensive patient with LV asymmetry, Bii – aortoseptal angle = 91 degrees.

aortic root dilatation and even in the context of obesity with raised hemidiaphragms secondary to increased visceral fat [41]. According to these findings, the diagnosis of HCM when HTN is present should not be based only on wall thickness [42].

With the use of CMR's unique tissue characterisation properties, one can introduce new discriminators for the assessment of hypertensive patients with HCM phenotypes—increased indexed LV mass, absence of systolic anterior motion of the anterior mitral valve leaflet/apparatus (SAM), and absence of mid-wall fibrosis are in favour to HHD [45].

The role of LVH on LVEF and myocardial shortening can be explored by using CMR strain measurements (**Figure 5**), with findings suggesting that LVEF is a poor index of systolic function in hypertensive patients in the setting of LVH [34].

End-diastolic and end-systolic endocardial and epicardial contours are drawn and propagated over the cardiac cycle commonly performed from two long-axis cines to calculate global longitudinal strain and strain rate or from the two chambers' short-axis cines to calculate radial strain. Feature tracking software extracts 3-d LV coordinates to allow measurement of LV strain and strain rate curves.

Hypertensive heart disease is usually considered a diastolic disorder since it often develops with preserved LVEF. Investigating the pathophysiology of LVH and the association with LV function using segmental engineering strain measurements derived from CMR indicate that end-diastolic wall thickness (EDWT), long axis shortening (LAS), and mid-wall circumferential fractional shortening (mFS) are linked to LVEF independently and significantly; this study supports findings from a previous CMR

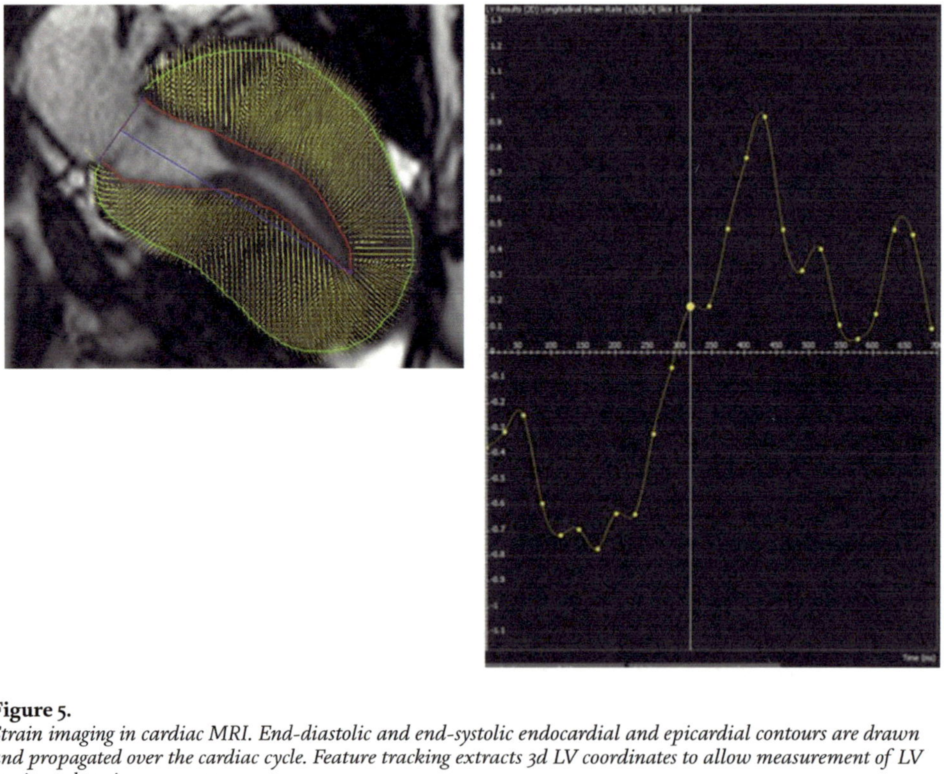

Figure 5.
Strain imaging in cardiac MRI. End-diastolic and end-systolic endocardial and epicardial contours are drawn and propagated over the cardiac cycle. Feature tracking extracts 3d LV coordinates to allow measurement of LV strain and strain rate curves.

study [32]. Increased EDWT and reduced myocardial fractional shortening lead to maintenance of absolute wall thickness (AWT) and thus preserved LVEF [34].

2.4 Hypertension and aortic disease

Aortic diseases are a major cause of cardiovascular morbidity and mortality [47]. Arterial stiffness is considered a major risk factor affecting the prognosis of hypertensive patients [48]. MRI can readily assess markers of aortic stiffness, pathological dilatation, vessel compliance, volume, and velocity of flow. Aortic stiffness is assessed by the measurement of distensibility using cross-sectional aortic area and diameter changes with the cardiac cycle and the simultaneous assessment of thoracic aortic pulse wave velocity (PWV) in the aortic arch; an increase in PWV may reflect increased aortic stiffness (**Figure 6**).

There are differences in myocardial intracellular and extracellular structure and a possible association with aortic function; there are differences in the prevalence of interstitial myocardial fibrosis, aortic distensibility and compliance, and myocardial circumferential strain between the varied hypertensive patterns, for example, concentric remodelling is linked to increased aortic stiffness [44].

Hypertension is often the common denominator in acute aortic syndrome (AAS) which encompasses a spectrum of entities from intramural hematoma, aortic dissection, and penetrating ulceration [49]. The treatment of AAS might include thoracic aortic stent grafting [50].

Given the above observations with respect to the 'selfish brain hypothesis', one might thus reflect on the stent graft positioning and the subsequent clinical follow-up of these patients who presented with a major vascular clinical consequence of chronic hypertension; if the left subclavian artery and thence left vertebral artery are covered by the stent-graft deployed to improve thoracic aortic dissection haemodynamics and/or prevent progressive aortic dilatation, this might have adverse consequences to hypertension control in the context of potential upstream deficiencies in the posterior cerebral circulation as described previously; thus, such positioning may potentially augment the very disease process that caused the AAS in the first place. This should be a subject of future work.

The prevalence of aortic coarctation (CoA) is ~4/10,000 live births [51] with arterial hypertension is considered a common complication (**Figure 7**) even post successful operative repair [52].

In both the above clinical entities, one might pay additional consideration to the cerebrovascular anatomy when the repair is planned for the reasons stated.

Furthermore, MRI can readily follow-up patients with chronic aortic dissection and also has the added advantage of being able to assess dissection flap dynamics which can adversely affect branch vessel perfusion. The MRI assessment of post-stent grafted aortas can be markedly affected by the nature and material of the graft material itself; some metallic artefacts can be catastrophic and therefore non-diagnostic in terms of image quality.

2.5 Concluding remarks and future perspectives

A thorough screening for secondary causes and asymptomatic organ damage is recommended for hypertensive patients according to hypertension ESC guidelines (**Figures 8–12**).

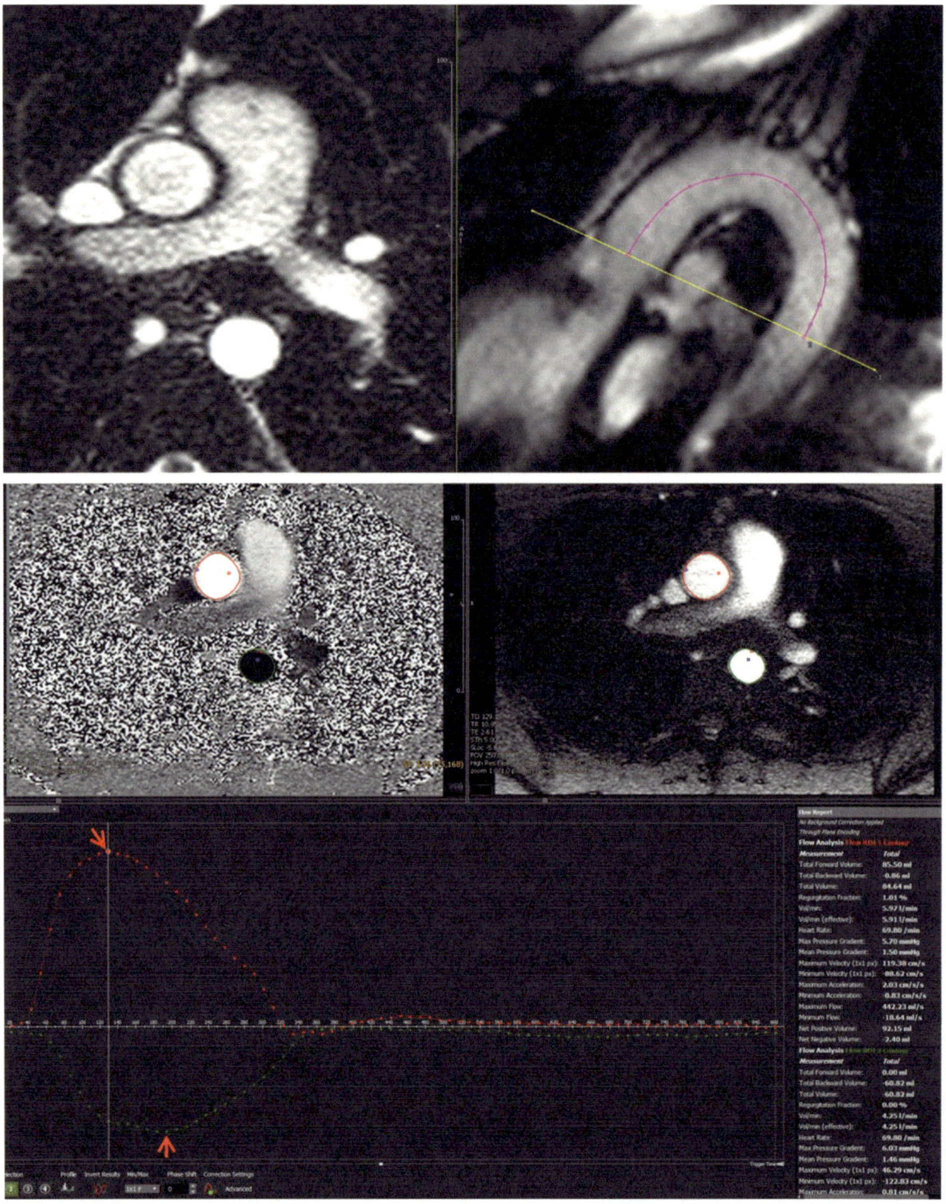

Figure 6.
Aortic arch assessment. Ascending and descending aortic areas are determined in end-diastole and end-systole (top left); this can give an indication of pathological dilatation and also of wall compliance. At the same cross-sectional level, the sampled aortic arch length is determined (top right) and breath-hold high temporal resolution phase-contrast CMR flow assessment is performed (middle); this enables generation of time - velocity/flow curves (bottom) from which can be derived additional data, such as the aortic pulse wave velocity. Red arrows point to the time (milliseconds) at peak velocity in the ascending aorta (red curve above) and the descending aorta (green curve below); then velocity (m/s) is the distance (mm)/time (ms).

As previously mentioned, echocardiography and abdominal/peripheral arterial ultrasound are used widely as first-line imaging tools even though the value of CMR is well-recognised [8].

CMR is known to be the gold standard non-invasive imaging technique for the assessment of cardiac anatomy and function, [10] with unique tissue characterisation properties, [11] and it does not require subjecting the patient to ionising radiation, is capable of imaging multiple organs and the vasculature with high diagnostic accuracy in a single session [9].

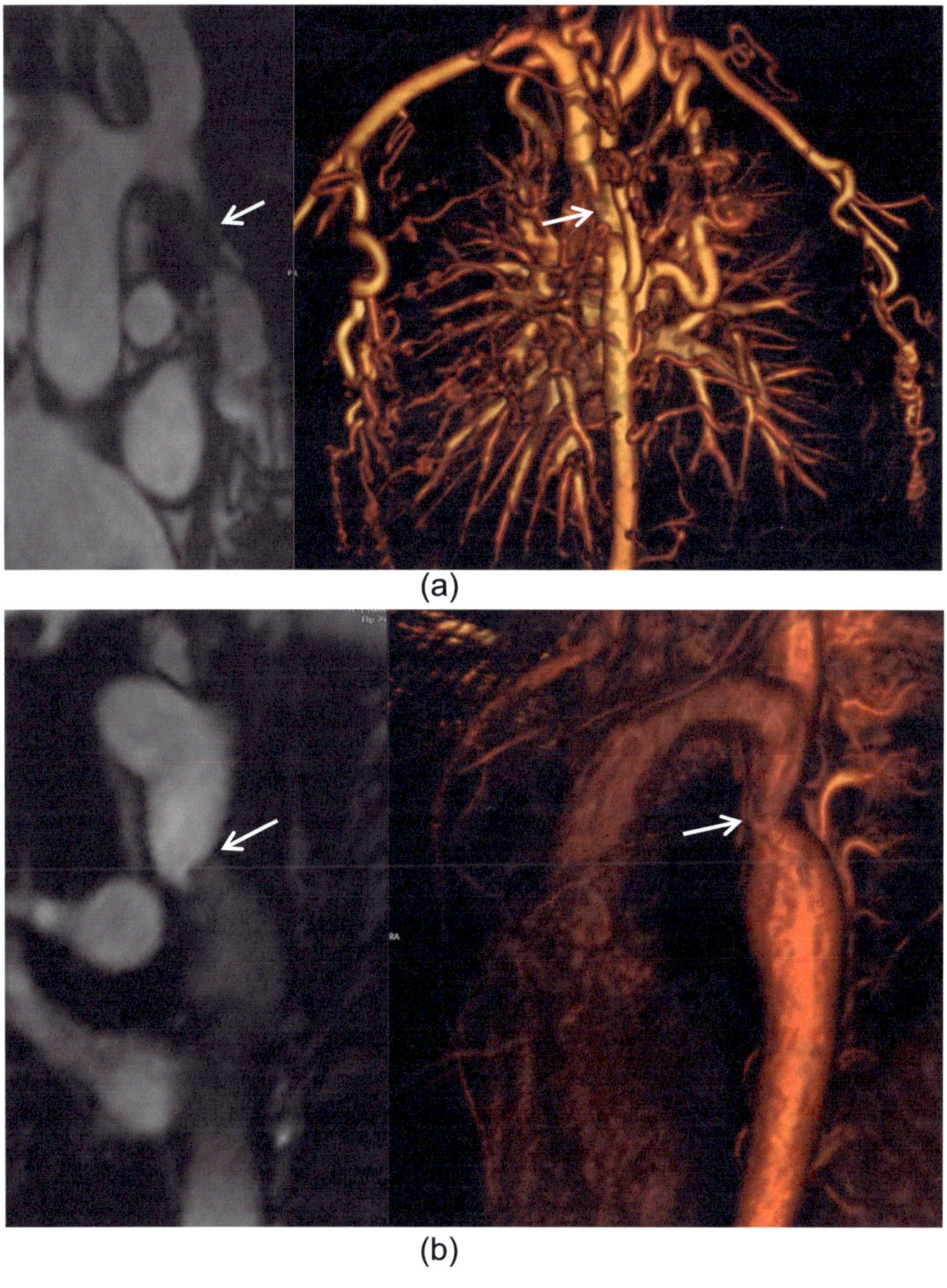

Figure 7.
Aortic interruption and severe coarctation. (a) – TrueFISP (left) and posterior view 3-dimensional MR angiography (right) showing a short aortic interruption (white arrows) with extensive lateral thoracic, internal mammary, and intercostal arterial collateralisation. (b) - TrueFISP (left) and left anterior oblique view 3-dimensional MR angiography (right) showing a focal tight aortic coarctation (white arrows) with a more notable membranous component at the level of the aortic isthmus with associated dilated intercostal arterial collateralisation.

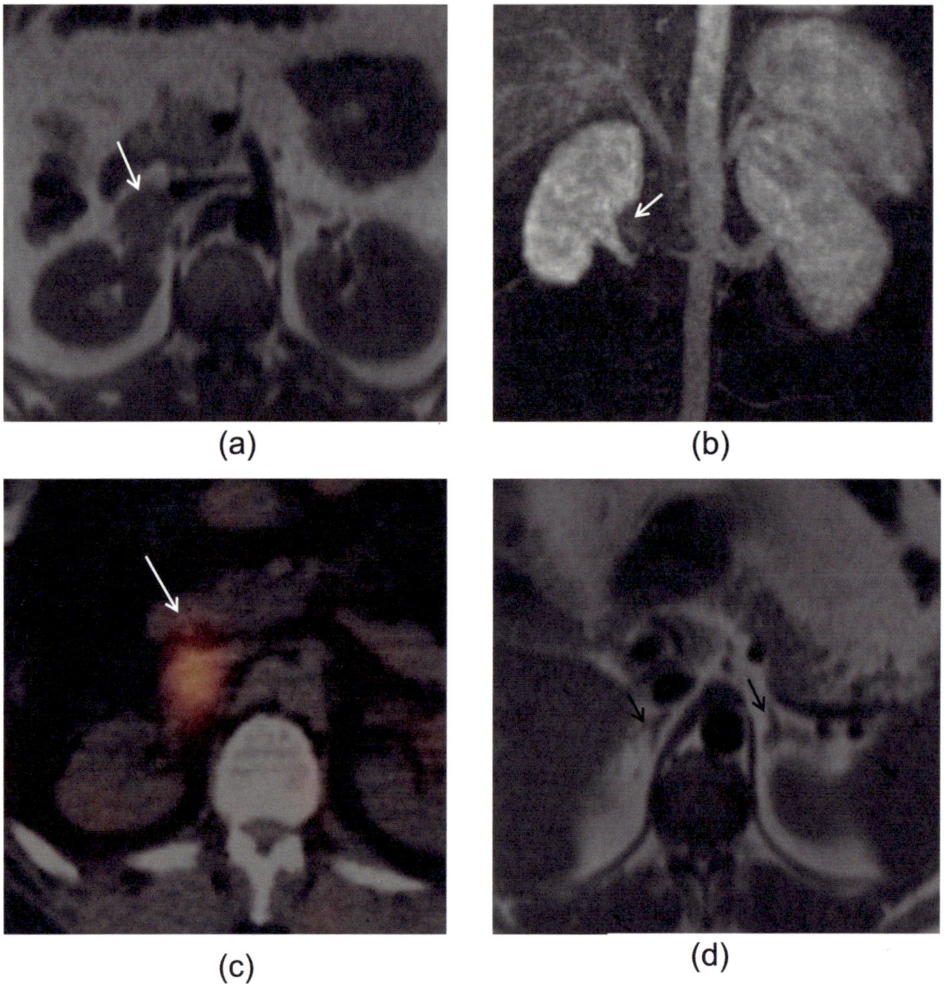

Figure 8.
Right-sided extra-adrenal phaeochromocytoma. (a) – Axial HASTE (Siemens). Half-Fourier Acquisition Single-shot Turbo spin Echo imaging. Well-defined, heterogenous soft tissue mass anterosuperior to the right renal hilum (white arrow). (b) – Multiphase gadolinium-enhanced angiography demonstrates homogenous enhancement (white arrow). (c) – MIBG (meta-iodo-benzyl-guanidine)-CT fusion imaging shows increased uptake within an extra-adrenal phaeochromocytoma (white arrow). (d) – Axial HASTE imaging shows bilateral normal adrenal glands (black arrows).

We advocate MRI as a safe and effective non-invasive screening imaging technique for hypertensive patients, using a comprehensive cardiac and non-cardiac protocol.

2.5.1 Implications for research and clinical practice

Ongoing studies are encouraged to investigate a) the relationship between the selfish brain hypothesis and hypertension (both childhood and young-onset hypertension), b) the relationship of these findings to the development of premature cerebrovascular disease or dementia especially in those who have their hypertension 'controlled' and in whom this may be too aggressive for them as individuals, c) the impact of hypertension on thoracic pathology, predicting adverse aortic remodelling

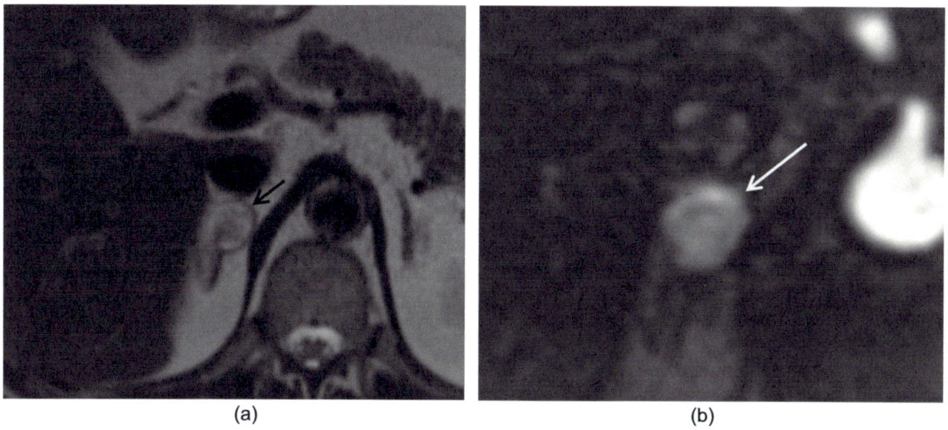

Figure 9.
Right adrenal phaeochromocytoma. (a) – Axial HASTE through the upper abdomen showing a heterogeneous, predominantly increased signal, well-defined soft tissue mass arising from the right adrenal gland (black arrow). (b) – Early phase axial angiography shows avid gadolinium enhancement of the mass (white arrow).

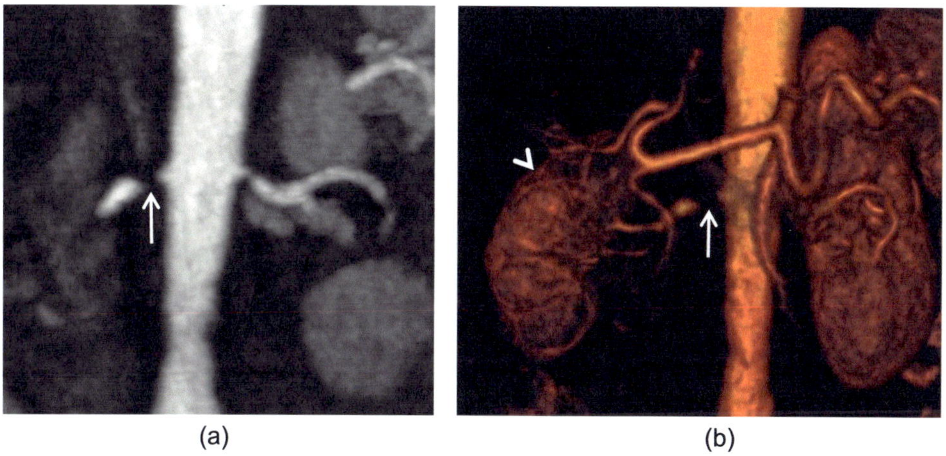

Figure 10.
Bilateral renal artery stenosis. Oblique coronal arterial phase gadolinium angiography showing a tight left renal artery stenosis and subtotal occlusion (white arrow) of the right renal artery (a) secondary to atherosclerosis, with associated right renal atrophy (white arrowhead) on 3-dimensional angiography (b). Note that the infrarenal abdominal aorta is atheromatous.

and the effect of the endovascular intervention on hypertensive patients with potentially important cerebrovascular variations, and d) the complex LV phenotype assessment by CMR and the effect of medical therapy on patterns of LV remodelling, LVH, and interstitial fibrosis, and thus the ultimate effect on patient prognosis.

If these findings were proven to be true, caution could be placed to the degree of BP reduction or nature of medication used in the hypertensive patient with VAH and incomplete posterior CoW and possibly avoid paradoxical adverse effects with treatment. From an investigational standpoint, the role of these cerebrovascular variants in the development of vascular dementia in hypertensive patients may need to be studied further. The future screening of cerebrovascular structure may require the screening of cerebrovascular anomalies in hypertensive patients, either via a Doppler

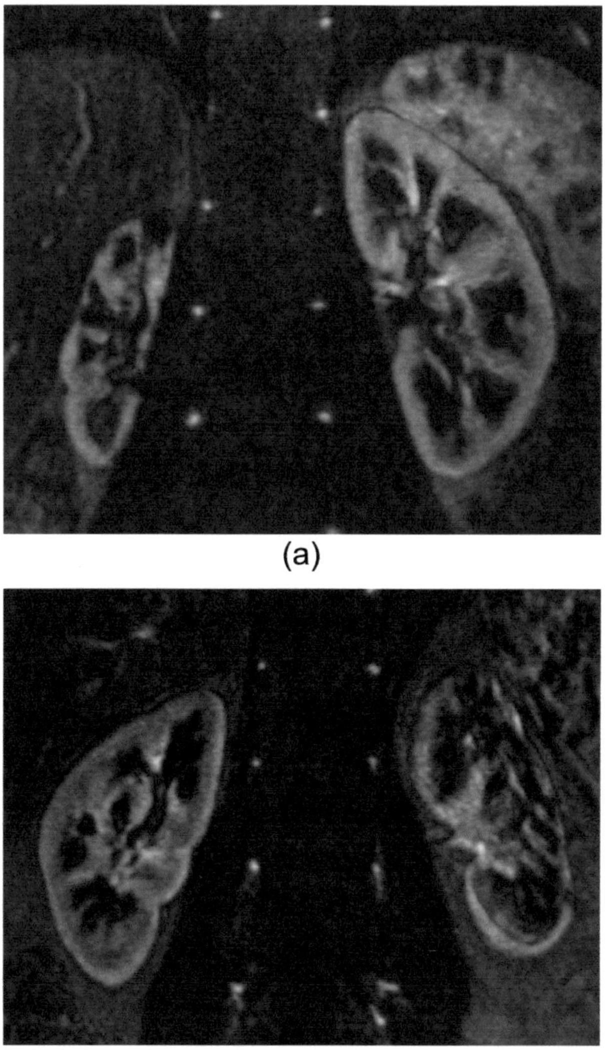

(a)

(b)

Figure 11.
Chronic unilateral renal atrophy with contralateral compensatory renal hypertrophy. Coronal early phase angiography shows severe right renal atrophy secondary to childhood reflux nephropathy (a) and severe left renal atrophy secondary to chronic pyelonephritis (b).

ultrasound or non-invasive angiographic imaging studies, such as computed tomographic angiography or magnetic resonance angiography.

Treatment of prehypertensive or borderline hypertensive patients with such anomalies may be directed towards using agents that mitigate sympathetic nerve activity such as angiotensin receptor blockers. This finding may also extrapolate to the treatment of acquired stenosis of the vertebrobasilar system from underlying atherosclerosis for which endovascular treatment is controversial.

Vertebral artery stenosis can be treated with stenting with good technical results, but whether it results in improved clinical outcomes is uncertain [53]. This study showed that stenting for vertebral stenosis has a much higher risk for intracranial

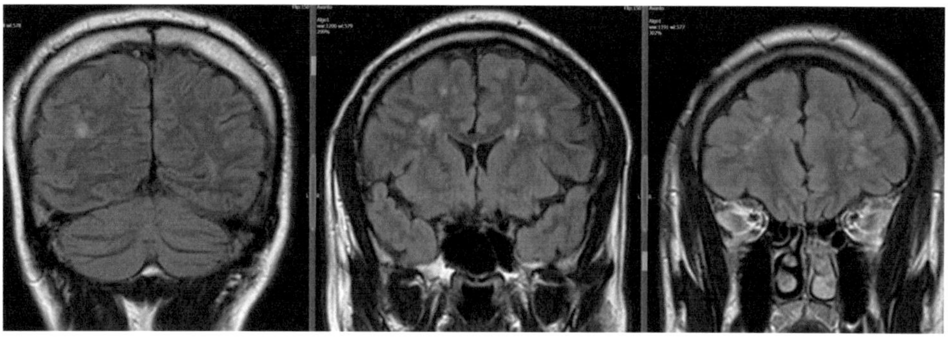

Figure 12.
Hypertensive cerebral microangiopathy. Coronal FLAIR imaging (Fluid-Attenuated Inversion Recovery is an inversion recovery sequence with a long inversion time; this removes the signal from the cerebrospinal fluid in the resulting images); shows patchy periventricular deep white matter high signal bilaterally in the frontal, parietal and occipital lobes in a patient with young-onset hypertension and cerebrovascular variation of the posterior circulation.

stenosis compared with extracranial stenosis; this pooled analysis did not show evidence of a benefit for stroke prevention for either treatment. In addition, the VIST trial compared the risks and benefits of vertebral angioplasty and stenting with best medical treatment alone for symptomatic vertebral artery stenosis; [54] this study also concluded that stenting in extracranial stenosis appears safe with low complication rates but that large phase 3 trials are required to determine whether stenting reduces stroke risk.

However, if the acquired stenosis or indeed congenital hypoplasia of the vertebral artery was found to be the cause of hypertension, vertebral stenting/angioplasty could be investigated for the possible benefit of an antihypertensive intervention.

Whether this pathologic mechanism is one of the unknown causes of essential hypertension and is more common than other previously proposed causes or a certain combination of pathological mechanisms underlie essential hypertension, remains to be definitively proven with longitudinal studies.

3. Summary

This chapter illustrates how the unique role of MRI can be used to comprehensively and non-invasively image patients with hypertension. In our institution, we have used such a protocol in those patients seen via a tertiary referral hypertension clinic for almost 10 years; such patients are generally difficult to treat/resistant hypertensives and young-onset hypertensive patients.

Patients who have sustained the consequences of a hypertensive insult, such as myocardial infarction, acute aortic dissection, cerebrovascular events, acute malignant hypertension, or pre-eclampsia, can also be assessed with MRI. Distinguishing between hypertensive heart disease and hypertrophic cardiomyopathy can be a particular challenge.

Importantly, we have also indicated how the 'selfish brain hypothesis' may play a vital role in the aetiology of 'essential hypertension'. Future studies are clearly needed and we suggest that MRI can play an increasingly pivotal role to help guide an efficient and bespoke therapeutic approach to patient management.

From a non-invasive imaging perspective, the hypertensive cohort is particularly interesting and challenging; a vast amount of important detail can be obtained in a single study. Nevertheless, we can take a step closer to uncovering the causes of the greatest non-communicable cause of human mortality and morbidity.

Acknowledgements

NIHR Cardiovascular Biomedical Research Unit, Bristol Heart Institute.

Jonathan Rodrigues, Elizabeth Robinson, Thomas Hinton, Julian Paton, Richard Wise, Laura Ratcliffe, Amy Burchell, and Angus Nightingale.

The MRI radiographers, Bristol Heart Institute. Bristol Heart Imaging Ltd for the kind research bursary awarded to Dr. Mitrousi.

Conflict of interest

The authors declare no conflict of interest.

Appendices and nomenclature

2D	two-dimensional
AAS	Acute aortic syndrome
AWT	Absolute wall thickness
BMI	Body mass index
BP	Blood pressure
CMR	Cardiovascular magnetic resonance imaging
CoA	Coarctation of the aorta
CT	Computed tomography
ECG	Electrocardiogram
EDWT	End -diastolic wall thickness
ESC	European Society of Cardiology
HCM	Hypertrophic cardiomyopathy
HHD	Hypertensive heart disease
HMOD	Hypertension mediated organ damage
HTN	Hypertension
ipCoW	Incomplete posterior circle of Willis
LAE	Left atrial enlargement
LAS	Long axis shortening
LV	Left ventricle
LVEF	Left ventricular ejection fraction
LVH	Left ventricular hypertrophy
LVM	Left ventricular mass
mFS	mid-wall circumferential fractional shortening
MR	Magnetic resonance
MRI	Magnetic resonance imaging
PWV	Pulse wave velocity
SAM	systolic anterior motion of mitral valve
VAH	Vertebral artery hypoplasia
VIST	Vertebral Artery Ischaemia Stenting Trial

Author details

Konstantina E. Mitrousi[1,2,3], Emma C. Hart[3], Mark C.K. Hamilton[1,4,5] and Nathan E. Manghat[1,3,4,5]*

1 NIHR Bristol Cardiovascular Biomedical Research Unit, Cardiac Magnetic Resonance Department, Bristol Heart Institute, University Hospitals Bristol NHS Foundation Trust, Bristol, UK

2 School of Physiology, Pharmacology and Neuroscience, Faculty of biomedical Sciences, University of Bristol, Bristol, UK

3 Cardionomics Research Group, Clinical Research and Imaging Centre, Bristol Heart Institute, University Hospitals Bristol NHS Foundation Trust, Bristol, UK

4 Department of Radiology, Bristol Royal Infirmary, University Hospitals Bristol NHS Foundation Trust, Bristol, UK

5 Bristol Heart Imaging Ltd, Bristol, UK

*Address all correspondence to: nathan.manghat@uhbw.nhs.uk

References

[1] Gull WW, Sutton HG. On the pathology of the morbid state commonly called chronic Bright's disease with contracted kidney, ("Arterio-capillary fibrosis."). Medico-Chirurgical Transactions. 1872;**55**:273-330

[2] Lim SS, Vos T, Flaxman AD, Danaei G, Shibuya K, Adair-Rohani H, et al. A comparative risk assessment of burden of disease and injury attributable to 67 risk factors and risk factor clusters in 21 regions, 1990-2010: A systematic analysis for the global burden of disease study 2010. Lancet. 2012;**380**(9859):2224-2260

[3] Gaziano TA, Bitton A, Anand S, Weinstein MC. Hypertension ISo. The global cost of nonoptimal blood pressure. Journal of Hypertension. 2009;**27**(7):1472-1477

[4] Sever PS, Poulter NR. A hypothesis for the pathogenesis of essential hypertension: The initiating factors. Journal of Hypertension. Supplement. 1989;7(1):S9-S12

[5] Ehret GB, Caulfield MJ. Genes for blood pressure: An opportunity to understand hypertension. European Heart Journal. 2013;**34**(13):951-961

[6] Elliott P, Marmot M, Dyer A, Joossens J, Kesteloot H, Stamler R, et al. The INTERSALT study: Main results, conclusions and some implications. Clinical and Experimental Hypertension. Part A. 1989;**11**(5-6):1025-1034

[7] Go AS, Bauman MA, Coleman King SM, Fonarow GC, Lawrence W, Williams KA, et al. An effective approach to high blood pressure control: A science advisory from the American Heart Association, the American College of Cardiology, and the Centers for Disease Control and Prevention. Journal of the American College of Cardiology. 2014;**63**(12):1230-1238

[8] Verdecchia P, Reboldi G, Angeli F. The 2020 International Society of Hypertension global hypertension pratice guidelines - Key messages and clinical considerations. Eur J Intern Med. 2020 Dec;**82**:1-6

[9] Burchell AE, Rodrigues JC, Charalambos M, Ratcliffe LE, Hart EC, Paton JF, et al. Comprehensive first-line magnetic resonance imaging in hypertension: Experience from a single-Center tertiary referral clinic. Journal of Clinical Hypertension (Greenwich, Conn.). 2017;**19**(1):13-22

[10] Keenan NG, Pennell DJ. CMR of ventricular function. Echocardiography. 2007 Feb;**24**(2):185-193

[11] Ferreira VM, Piechnik SK, Robson MD, Neubauer S, Karamitsos TD. Myocardial tissue characterization by magnetic resonance imaging novel applications of T1 and T2 mapping. Journal of Thoracic Imaging. 2014 May;**29**(3):147-154

[12] Biglino G, Steeden JA, Baker C, Schievano S, Taylor AM, Parker KH, et al. A non-invasive clinical application of wave intensity analysis based on ultrahigh temporal resolution phase-contrast cardiovascular magnetic resonance. Journal of Cardiovascular Magnetic Resonance. 2012;**14**:57

[13] Obokata M, Nagata Y, Wu VC, Kado Y, Kurabayashi M, Otsuji Y, et al. Direct comparison of cardiac magnetic resonance feature tracking and 2D/3D echocardiography speckle tracking for evaluation of global left

ventricular strain. European Heart Journal Cardiovascular Imaging. 2016;**17**(5):525-532

[14] Mancia G, Grassi G. The autonomic nervous system and hypertension. Circulation Research. 2014;**114**(11):1804-1814

[15] Cates MJ, Steed PW, Abdala AP, Langton PD, Paton JF. Elevated vertebrobasilar artery resistance in neonatal spontaneously hypertensive rats. Journal of Applied Physiology (1985). 2011; **111**(1): 149-156

[16] Dickinson CJ, Thomason AD. Vertebral and internal carotid arteries in relation to hypertension and cerebrovascular disease. Lancet. 1959;**2**(7090):46-48

[17] Paton JF, Dickinson CJ, Mitchell G. Harvey Cushing and the regulation of blood pressure in giraffe, rat and man: Introducing 'Cushing's mechanism. Experimental Physiology. 2009;**94**(1):11-17

[18] Hart EC. Human hypertension, sympathetic activity and the selfish brain. Experimental Physiology. 2016;**101**(12):1451-1462

[19] Manghat N, Robinson E, Mitrousi K, Rodrigues J, Hinton T, Paton J, et al. Cerebrovascular variants and the role of the selfish brain in young onset hypertension. Hypertension. 2022 March 16:HYPERTENSIONAHA12118612 *In Press*. DOI: 0.1161/HYPER-TENSIONAHA.121.18612. [online ahead of print]

[20] Rodrigues JCL, Jaring MFR, Werndle MC, Mitrousi K, Lyen SM, Nightingale AK, et al. Repaired coarctation of the aorta, persistent arterial hypertension and the selfish brain. Journal of Cardiovascular Magnetic Resonance. 2019;**21**(1):68

[21] Koren MJ, Devereux RB, Casale PN, Savage DD, Laragh JH. Relation of left ventricular mass and geometry to morbidity and mortality in uncomplicated essential hypertension. Annals of Internal Medicine. 1991;**114**(5): 345-352

[22] Kannel WB, Doyle JT, Mcnamara PM, Quickenton P, Gordon T. Precursors of sudden coronary death. Factors related to the incidence of sudden death. Circulation. 1975;**51**(4):606-613

[23] McLenachan JM, Dargie HJ. Left ventricular hypertrophy as a factor in arrhythmias and sudden death. American Journal of Hypertension. 1989; **2**(2 Pt 1):128-131

[24] Levy D, Larson MG, Vasan RS, Kannel WB, Ho KK. The progression from hypertension to congestive heart failure. Journal of the American Medical Association. 1996;**275**(20):1557-1562

[25] Fox ER, Alnabhan N, Penman AD, Butler KR, Taylor HA, Skelton TN, et al. Echocardiographic left ventricular mass index predicts incident stroke in African Americans. Stroke. 2007 Oct;**38**(10):2686-2691

[26] Casale PN, Devereux RB, Kligfield P, Eisenberg RR, Miller DH, Chaudhary BS, et al. Electrocardiographic detection of left ventricular hypertrophy: Development and prospective validation of improved criteria. Journal of the American College of Cardiology. 1985;**6**(3):572-580

[27] Landsberg L, Aronne LJ, Beilin LJ, Burke V, Igel LI, Lloyd-Jones D, et al. Obesity-related hypertension: Pathogenesis, cardiovascular risk, and treatment--a position paper of the Obesity Society and the American Society of Hypertension. Obesity (Silver Spring). 2013;**21**(1):8-24

[28] Rodrigues JC, McIntyre B, Dastidar AG, Lyen SM, Ratcliffe LE, Burchell AE, et al. The effect of obesity on electrocardiographic detection of hypertensive left ventricular hypertrophy: Recalibration against cardiac magnetic resonance. Journal of Human Hypertension. 2016;**30**(3):197-203

[29] Hancock EW, Deal BJ, Mirvis DM, Okin P, Kligfield P, Gettes LS, et al. AHA/ACCF/HRS recommendations for the standardization and interpretation of the electrocardiogram: Part V: Electrocardiogram changes associated with cardiac chamber hypertrophy: A scientific statement from the American Heart Association electrocardiography and arrhythmias committee, council on clinical cardiology; the American College of Cardiology Foundation; and the Heart Rhythm Society. Endorsed by the International Society for Computerized Electrocardiology. Journal of the American College of Cardiology. 2009;**53**(11):992-1002

[30] Okin PM, Devereux RB, Nieminen MS, Jern S, Oikarinen L, Viitasalo M, et al. Electrocardiographic strain pattern and prediction of cardiovascular morbidity and mortality in hypertensive patients. Hypertension. 2004;**44**(1):48-54

[31] Querejeta R, Varo N, López B, Larman M, Artiñano E, Etayo JC, et al. Serum carboxy-terminal propeptide of procollagen type I is a marker of myocardial fibrosis in hypertensive heart disease. Circulation. 2000;**101**(14): 1729-1735

[32] Palmon LC, Reichek N, Yeon SB, Clark NR, Brownson D, Hoffman E, et al. Intramural myocardial shortening in hypertensive left ventricular hypertrophy with normal pump function. Circulation. 1994;**89**(1):122-131

[33] Rodrigues JC, Amadu AM, Ghosh Dastidar A, McIntyre B, Szantho GV, Lyen S, et al. ECG strain pattern in hypertension is associated with myocardial cellular expansion and diffuse interstitial fibrosis: A multi-parametric cardiac magnetic resonance study. European Heart Journal Cardiovascular Imaging. 2017;**18**(4):441-450

[34] Rodrigues JC, Rohan S, Dastidar AG, Trickey A, Szantho G, Ratcliffe LE, et al. The relationship between left Ventricular Wall thickness, myocardial shortening, and ejection fraction in hypertensive heart disease: Insights from cardiac magnetic resonance imaging. Journal of Clinical Hypertension (Greenwich, Conn.). 2016;**18**(11):1119-1127

[35] Movahed MR, Saito Y. Obesity is associated with left atrial enlargement, E/a reversal and left ventricular hypertrophy. Experimental and Clinical Cardiology. 2008;**13**(2):89-91

[36] Weber MA, Schiffrin EL, White WB, Mann S, Lindholm LH, Kenerson JG, et al. Clinical practice guidelines for the management of hypertension in the community: A statement by the American Society of Hypertension and the International Society of Hypertension. Journal of Clinical Hypertension (Greenwich, Conn.). 2014;**16**(1):14-26

[37] Tsang TS, Abhayaratna WP, Barnes ME, Miyasaka Y, Gersh BJ, Bailey KR, et al. Prediction of cardiovascular outcomes with left atrial size: Is volume superior to area or diameter? Journal of the American College of Cardiology. 2006;**47**(5):1018-1023

[38] Waggoner AD, Adyanthaya AV, Quinones MA, Alexander JK. Left atrial enlargement. Echocardiographic assessment of electrocardiographic criteria. Circulation. 1976;**54**(4):553-557

[39] Rodrigues JC, Erdei T, Dastidar AG, McIntyre B, Burchell AE, Ratcliffe LE, et al. Electrocardiographic detection of hypertensive left atrial enlargement in the presence of obesity: re-calibration against cardiac magnetic resonance. Journal of Human Hypertension. 2017;**31**(3):212-219

[40] Ganau A, Devereux RB, Roman MJ, de Simone G, Pickering TG, Saba PS, et al. Patterns of left ventricular hypertrophy and geometric remodeling in essential hypertension. Journal of the American College of Cardiology. 1992;**19**(7):1550-1558

[41] Tuseth N, Cramariuc D, Rieck AE, Wachtell K, Gerdts E. Asymmetric septal hypertrophy - a marker of hypertension in aortic stenosis (a SEAS substudy). Blood Pressure. 2010;**19**(3):140-144

[42] Rodrigues JC, Amadu AM, Dastidar AG, Hassan N, Lyen SM, Lawton CB, et al. Prevalence and predictors of asymmetric hypertensive heart disease: Insights from cardiac and aortic function with cardiovascular magnetic resonance. European Heart Journal Cardiovascular Imaging. 2016;**17**(12):1405-1413

[43] Dweck MR, Joshi S, Murigu T, Gulati A, Alpendurada F, Jabbour A, et al. Left ventricular remodeling and hypertrophy in patients with aortic stenosis: Insights from cardiovascular magnetic resonance. Journal of Cardiovascular Magnetic Resonance. 2012;**14**:50

[44] Rodrigues JC, Amadu AM, Dastidar AG, Szantho GV, Lyen SM, Godsave C, et al. Comprehensive characterisation of hypertensive heart disease left ventricular phenotypes. Heart. 2016;**102**(20):1671-1679

[45] Rodrigues JC, Rohan S, Ghosh Dastidar A, Harries I, Lawton CB, Ratcliffe LE, et al. Hypertensive heart disease versus hypertrophic cardiomyopathy: Multi-parametric cardiovascular magnetic resonance discriminators when end-diastolic wall thickness >/= 15 mm. European Radiology. 2017;**27**(3):1125-1135

[46] Elliott PM, Anastasakis A, Borger MA, Borggrefe M, Cecchi F, Charron P, et al. 2014 ESC guidelines on diagnosis and management of hypertrophic cardiomyopathy: The task force for the diagnosis and Management of Hypertrophic Cardiomyopathy of the European Society of Cardiology (ESC). European Heart Journal. 2014;**35**(39):2733-2779

[47] Arturo Evangelista Frank A. Flachskampf, Raimund Erbel, Francesco Antonini-Canterin, Charalambos Vlachopoulos , Guido Rocchi, Rosa Sicari, Petros Nihoyannopoulos, Jose Zamorano, European Association of Echocardiography. Echocardiography in aortic diseases: EAE recommendations for clinical practice. Eur J Echocardiogr. 2010 sep;**11**(8):645-658

[48] Safar ME. Arterial stiffness as a risk factor for clinical hypertension. Nature Reviews. Cardiology. 2018;**15**(2):97-105

[49] Bossone E, Eagle KA. Epidemiology and management of aortic disease: Aortic aneurysms and acute aortic syndromes. Nature Reviews. Cardiology. 2021;**18**(5):331-348

[50] Mussa FF, Horton JD, Moridzadeh R, Nicholson J, Trimarchi S, Eagle KA. Acute aortic dissection and intramural hematoma: A systematic review. Journal of the American Medical Association. 2016;**316**(7):754-763

[51] Hoffman JI, Kaplan S. The incidence of congenital heart disease. Journal of the American College of Cardiology. 2002 Jun 19;**39**(12):1890-1900

[52] Toro-Salazar OH, Steinberger J, Thomas W, Rocchini AP, Carpenter B, Moller JH. Long-term follow-up of patients after coarctation of the aorta repair. The American Journal of Cardiology. 2002;**89**(5):541-547

[53] Markus HS, Harshfield EL, Compter A, Kuker W, Kappelle LJ, Clifton A, et al. Stenting for symptomatic vertebral artery stenosis: A preplanned pooled individual patient data analysis. Lancet Neurology. 2019 Jul;**18**(7):666-673

[54] Markus HS, Larsson SC, Kuker W, Schulz UG, Ford I, Rothwell PM, et al. Stenting for symptomatic vertebral artery stenosis: The vertebral artery ischaemia stenting trial. Neurology. 2017;**89**(12):1229-1236

Chapter 4

Mechanism of Development of Arterial Hypertension Associated with the Exchange of Level Vitamin D

Sona Gahramanova

Abstract

Arterial hypertension (AH) is one of the most chronic and fatal disorders in the world, the main risk factors for which are age, hereditary predisposition, race, tobacco use, high salt intake, etc., as well as low vitamin D. In the last 10 years, there has been an increasing interest in the extraosseous effects of vitamin D. Being a hormone-like vitamin, it participates in many vital processes of the body. Its level is closely related to various metabolic disorders, diseases of the cardiovascular system (CVS), arterial hypertension (AH), diabetes mellitus, the immune system, cancer, etc. Vitamin D improves vascular endothelial function, due to which it has a vasoprotective effect, improves blood pressure, reduces vascular and myocardial remodeling, reduces the risk of left ventricular hypertrophy, slows down fibrosis, reduces the risk of atherosclerosis, reduces insulin resistance and inflammation, and improves immunity. It has been proven that vitamin D has an inverse relationship with renin, it reduces the expression of the renin gene. At a normal level of vitamin D, the concentration of renin and aldosterone II decreases, which has a positive effect on the course of hypertension.

Keywords: arterial hypertension, blood pressure, vitamin D, receptors, genes

1. Introduction

As we know, diseases of the circulatory system occupy the leading place among diseases leading to disability and mortality of the population. Arterial hypertension (AH) today remains the main risk factor for cardiovascular diseases (CVD).

Hypertension is not just a chronic increase in blood pressure (BP), it is a poly etiological disease, which is based on hemodynamic, neurohumoral, and metabolic disorders, leading to serious consequences (atherosclerosis, myocardial infarction, cerebrovascular diseases—cerebral strokes, heart failure), impairs memory, vision, and negatively affects renal function, leading to renal failure.

Today, an asymptomatic increase in blood pressure is increasingly manifested, which indicates a greater likelihood of the prevalence of hypertension. Therefore, for early diagnosis of hypertension, frequent measurement of blood pressure is recommended for persons without clinical complaints of high blood pressure.

The term "arterial hypertension" refers to the syndrome of persistent elevation of systolic blood pressure (SBP) $\geq$ 140 mm Hg and/or diastolic blood pressure (DBP) $\geq$90 mm Hg, which, depending on etio-pathological factors, manifests itself as primary hypertension (essential) or proceeds as a secondary condition. No less important in the pathogenesis of essential hypertension is a change in the arterial wall—a decrease and then a complete loss of the contractile function of the muscle layer and vascular endothelium, as well as atherosclerotic changes [1].

The main pathogenetic factor in the development of hypertension is the activation of the sympatho-adrenal (SAS) and renin-angiotensin-aldosterone system (RAAS)—which, as a rule, is the most powerful neurohormonal system of the body, the activation of which can result in the development of coronary heart disease, heart failure (HF). Heredity, diabetes mellitus (DM), the presence of metabolic syndrome, unhealthy diet, increased consumption of sodium chloride (more than 6 g of table salt per day), obesity (components of the RAAS are produced in the adipocytes of adipose tissue), lack of physical activity (physical inactivity), psycho-emotional exercise, smoking, excessive drinking, and according to recent data, low levels of vitamin D are also risk factors for the development of hypertension. Along with a large number of studies proving the role of vitamin D in reducing SBP and DBP, there are other works confirming the insignificant role of vitamin D deficiency in the pathogenesis of hypertension [2]. The increased blood pressure or the risk of hypertension is hypothesized to be due in part to the patients' baseline vitamin D levels, sample size, and length of follow-up. It should also be borne in mind that diseases such as diabetes mellitus, kidney disease, underlying cardiovascular disease can affect the physiological mechanisms of vitamin D action on blood pressure. This explains the significant differences between individual patients in the values of vitamin D [3–5].

2. Biological role of vitamin D

Vitamin D was discovered in the early 1920s (1922) of the twentieth century by Windaus. The work of recent years indicates that the biological role of vitamin D is not limited to the effect only on calcium metabolism, but also plays an important role in maintaining the immune and endocrine system, metabolic processes, cardiovascular and cerebrovascular health, and also significantly reduces the risk of developing tumors, tuberculosis, rheumatoid arthritis, etc. Biological functions of vitamin D are shown in **Figure 1**.

Since the middle of the twentieth century, vitamin D deficiency (D-deficiency) has acquired not only medical, but also medico-social significance. The causes of D-deficiency are demographic changes—an aging population, an increase in geriatric pathology, unbalanced nutrition, a low level of physical activity, insufficient exposure to the sun, and a decrease in insolation. Receptors to calcitriol are found not only in enterocytes and bones, but also in the kidneys, neurocytes, pancreas, myocytes of striated and smooth muscles, bone marrow cells, immunocompetent cells, and genitals (**Figure 1**). Therefore, the functional role of the hormone vitamin is not limited to participation in the regulation of calcium-phosphorus metabolism. A lot of information has been accumulated on the specific effects of calcitriol that are not related to its calcitropic activity: suppression of hyperproliferation, carcinogenesis, influence on cell growth and development, modulation of apoptosis, regulation of autoimmunity through effects on T- and B-lymphocytes, macrophages [6, 7].

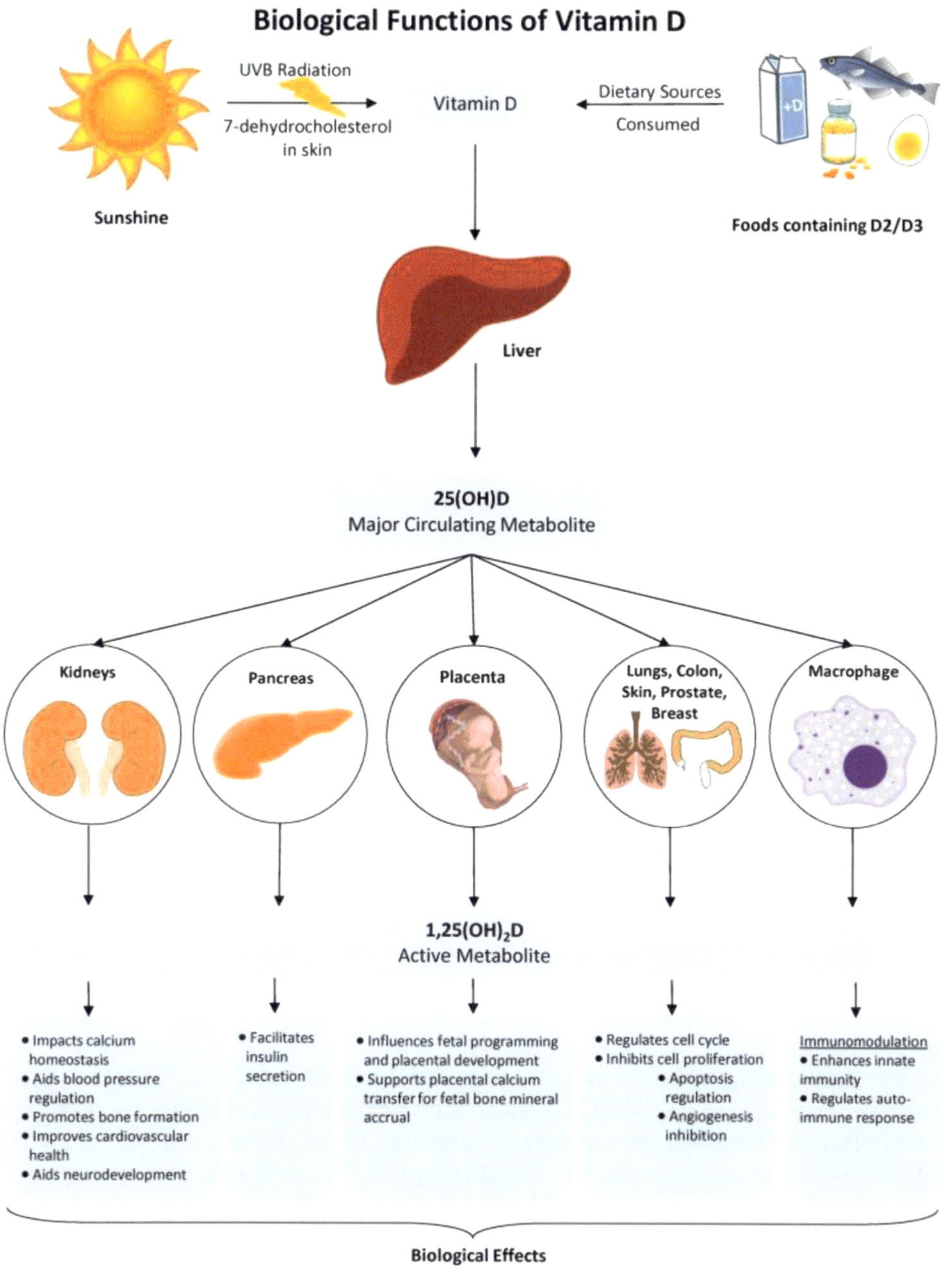

Figure 1.
Biological functions of vitamin D (based on the figure from the article Laura Lockaua Stephanie, A. Atkinson. Vitamin D's role in health and disease: How does the present inform our understanding of the past? International journal of paleopathology, vol. 23, December 2018, pages 6–14).

With sufficient and regular insolation, a person's need for vitamin D is fully met by photochemical synthesis in the skin. This is why vitamin D3 is called the "sunshine vitamin." It is the photochemical stages that are decisive in the activity of the D-hormonal system. Dietary source of vitamin D plays only a compensatory role in cases of endogenous vitamin deficiency.

Vitamin D3 has both endogenous origin (synthesized in the skin under the influence of ultraviolet rays from the precursor of 7-dehydrocholesterol) and exogenous (from animal food: fish oil, liver, egg yolk). All other food products are practically devoid of vitamin D. In this regard, in a number of countries it is specially added to some products, for example, milk, fruit juices, margarine. On the contrary, vitamin D2 (ergocalciferol) enters the body only with plant foods (bread, milk) and in very small quantities [8].

Endogenous vitamin D3 and its metabolites from the skin and/or vitamin D3 supplied with food, with the help of a transport D-binding protein, enter the subsequent stages in the liver, kidneys, where the hormone calcitriol is synthesized. 1,25 (OH) 2 D3- calcitriol or dihydroxycholecalciferol is a hormone similar to other steroid hormones, which controls about 1500–2000 genes through VDR receptors, including genes involved in the production of renin, insulin, growth, and proliferation of smooth muscle cells vessels and cardiomyocytes, and is involved in many processes. Vitamin D receptors, which are involved in the formation of vitamin D, are found in the cardiomyocytes of the ventricles of the heart. It has been proven that a decrease in the activity of vitamin D receptors can lead to remodeling of cardiomyocytes. The introduction of the active form of vitamin D helps to reduce this remodeling due to the effect on the functional, anatomical, molecular, and genetic aspects of hypertrophy and dysfunction of cardiomyocytes. A study conducted on newly diagnosed treatment-naïve hypertensive patients showed that hypovitaminosis D was a strong predictor of increased left ventricular mass index [9].

According to the Institute of Medicine (IOM), vitamin D deficiency is defined as circulating 25-hydroxyvitamin D (25[OH]D) level < 50 nmol/L based on the optimal concentration for skeletal health [10].

3. Role of vitamin D in pathophysiology and development of hypertension

Vitamin D has the potential to affect blood pressure through several mechanisms including those involving the renin-angiotensin-aldosterone system (RAAS), the endothelium, and vascular smooth muscle. Chronic treatment with active vitamin D compounds modulates vascular tone, reduces blood pressure and cyclooxegenase-1, and increases endothelial dysfunction and reactive oxygen species (ROS) in rats [11].

The association of arterial hypertension with low insolation and low levels of vitamin D in the blood serum was noted back in the 1990s of the twentieth century. In 1980, it was found that impaired calcium homeostasis, including hyperparathyroidism, may be involved in the mechanism of the development of hypertension and proved a significant decrease in calcium excretion in patients with hypertension compared with the control group. In 1988, Lind et al. [12] conducted a placebo-controlled study evaluating the effect of 0.5 μg alpha-calcidol, a vitamin D analog, on blood pressure in hypertensive patients with impaired glucose tolerance (mean age 62 years, n = 26) for 12 weeks. They found a significant decrease in SBP/DBP from 171/95 to 150/88 mm Hg after treatment.

The prevalence of vitamin D deficiency is directly related to higher latitudes due to less intense UVB radiation, colder climates due to less skin exposure, and darker skin as it interferes with UVB penetration and decreases vitamin D production [13]. The fact that a higher EH frequency is observed in winter in people living at higher latitudes and in people with deep skin pigmentation living far from the equator suggests that vitamin D deficiency may contribute to an increased prevalence of arterial hypertension. To test this hypothesis, Krause et al. [14] used ultraviolet radiation to treat patients with untreated mild arterial hypertension (AH) and vitamin D deficiency. These researchers found that UV radiation increased 25 (OH) D levels and lowered blood pressure in patients with vitamin D deficiency with AH. Since 1998, this discovery has generated significant research interest in the relationship between vitamin D deficiency and AH.

The relationship between the concentration of calcitriol in the blood serum and the level of blood pressure has been proven. When analyzing data from the NHANES III (National Health and Nutrition Examination Survey), an inverse significant relationship between the content of vitamin D3 and blood pressure indicators was revealed: in the group with a content of 25 (OH) D3 > 85.7 nmol/L, the levels of systolic blood pressure (SBP) and diastolic blood pressure (DBP) were 3, 0, and 1.6 mm Hg lower than in gr. with a content of 25 (OH) D3 < 40 nmol/L, respectively [15].

Hypertension is an age-dependent complex common feature with interactions between environmental and genetic factors. The incidence rises sharply in men over 45 and in women over 55. Vitamin D deficiency can be considered a risk factor for the development of arterial hypertension, contributing to a shift in the balance between vasodilator and vasoconstrictor factors in favor of vasoconstriction, which leads to the development of hypertension in people, mainly middle-aged people. Therefore, it is believed that an adequately selected dose of vitamin D, contributing to the normalization of the level of 25 (OH) D in the blood, effectively lowers blood pressure in patients with arterial hypertension with vitamin D deficiency. The authors concluded that when people have a stable balance between vasodilatory and vasoconstrictor factors in vitamin D deficiency, vitamin D supplementation has minimal effect on BP in a relatively short period. And when people have an unstable balance between vasodilating and vasoconstrictor factors, vitamin D deficiency becomes a risk factor contributing to the development of hypertension at age > 45 years; In this case, vitamin D supplementation can lower blood pressure [16]. Thus, vitamin D deficiency does not play an important role in the normal regulation of blood pressurc, and its excess may have a minimal effect on blood pressure in persons with normotension under the age of 45 years.

Genetic analyses, specifically Mendelian randomization studies, found that individuals with genetically lower serum 25(OH)D levels have an increased incidence of hypertension, implying that vitamin D deficiency may play a role in the development of hypertension. The largest genetic analysis included 142,255 individuals and found that a 10% increase in genetically determined 25(OH)D concentration was associated with a 0.37 mmHg lower systolic pressure (95% CI, 0.003–0.73 mmHg lower) [17].

Most of the main studies showed that BP was inversely and significantly correlated with the level of 25 (OH) D. Burgaz et al. conducted a meta-analysis including four prospective studies and 14 crossover studies to assess the association between circulating 25 (OH) D levels and arterial hypertension. They found an inverse relationship between serum 25 (OH) D concentration and arterial hypertensive incidence [18]. Forman JP et al. [19] conducted a four-beam, double-blind, placebo-controlled, randomized study in 283 black Americans (mean age of 51 years) to evaluate the effect of 1000, 2000, and 4000 IU of vitamin D per day or placebo on blood pressure for a period of 3 months. Baseline 25 (OH) D levels were about 16 ng/ml. The baseline mean blood pressure (122/78 mm Hg) was relatively lower because only 50% of the participants were hypertensive and 40% were taking antihypertensive drugs. The difference between systolic blood pressure at the beginning of the study and after 3 months was +1.7 mm Hg in the placebo group, −0.66 mm Hg in the group with 1000 IU of vitamin D, −3.44 mm Hg in the group with 2000 IU of vitamin D, and – 4.0 mm Hg In the group with vitamin D 4000 IU (−1.4 mm Hg for every 1000 IU additional intake of vitamin D, p = 0.04). For every 1 ng/ml increase in 25 (OH) D levels, a significant 0.2 mmHg reduction in systolic blood pressure was found.

4. Role of vitamin D in the regulation of RAAS and sympathetic activation

In the regulation of blood pressure, electrolyte homeostasis, the renin-angiotensin-aldosterone system (RAAS) plays an important role. An increase in the activity of the RAAS is considered as the most important link in the pathogenesis of hypertension. It is known that some antihypertensive drugs regulate blood pressure by affecting the renin-angiotensin-aldosterone system (RAAS). This system regulates plasma electrolyte levels, vascular resistance, and fluid volume homeostasis. Renin is an enzyme produced by the cells of the juxtaglomerular apparatus in the nephrons of the kidneys. Its synthesis is activated by renal hypoperfusion and activation of the sympathetic nervous system. Renin converts the angiotensinogen produced in the liver into angiotensin I, which is converted into angiotensin II under the influence of the angiotensin-converting enzyme (ACE) expressed in the lungs. Angiotensin 2, binding to its receptor, has a biological effect on the activity of the brain, heart, kidneys, peripheral vessels, and adrenal glands (**Figure 2**). The relationship between vitamin D levels and RAAS activity has been demonstrated in numerous studies [20, 21].

Numerous epidemiological studies have shown the association of low vitamin D levels with an increased risk of arterial hypertension [20]. Experimental studies in mice with damage to vitamin D receptors showed increased activity of renin and circulating angiotensin II, which led to arterial hypertension, which could be reduced by blocking the RAAS [21–23]. In other studies, mice that were unable to activate vitamin D in the body due to 1-alpha hydroxylase deficiency exhibited a similar phenotype to animals that lacked vitamin D receptors [24]. In this case, the addition of vitamin D led to a complete change in the phenotype, which confirms the role of vitamin D in the activation of the RAAS and in the development of arterial hypertension. Other animal experiments have demonstrated the ability of vitamin D to increase the concentration of intracellular calcium, which led to a decrease in renin secretion by juxtaglomerular cells [25].

Some studies have shown that vitamin D clearly inhibits renin biosynthesis and RAAS activity. Administration of an AT II receptor antagonist or angiotensin-converting enzyme (ACE inhibitor) inhibitor prevented or neutralized the above disorders. Later it was found that the activation of vitamin D receptors helps to reduce left ventricular hypertrophy (LVH) and prevents the activation of some components of the RAAS. An interesting fact is that the suppression of renin secretion by vitamin D through the activation of its receptors occurs independently of calcium homeostasis and disturbances in water-salt metabolism. In obese subjects with vitamin D deficiency, it found that treatment with ergocalciferol reduced kidney-specific RAS activity and blood pressure [26–28]. Thus, RAS activation may be a mechanism linking vitamin D with incident hypertension.

However, in another study, systemic RAS activity measured by plasma renin activity did not change significantly following 8 weeks of treatment with vitamin D (from 0.34 ± 0.37 ng/ml/hour to 0.36 ± 0.44 ng/ml/hour; p-value = 0.72) or placebo (0.42 ± 0.44 ng/ml/hour to 0.44 ± 0.80 ng/ml/hour, p-value = 0.85).

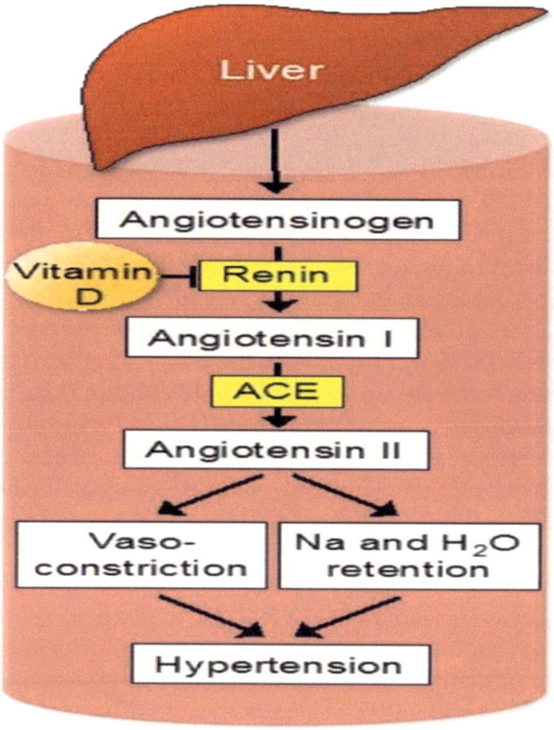

Figure 2.
Role of vitamin D in the regulation of RAAS.

Similarly, serum angiotensin II levels did not change significantly after 8 weeks of treatment with either ergocalciferol or placebo. There was no significant change in mean 24-hour systolic blood pressure or other ambulatory measurements following treatment with either ergocalciferol or placebo [29]. In this placebo-controlled, randomized study, it was found that in obese patients with vitamin D deficiency without arterial hypertension, the correction of vitamin D level does not affect the level of blood pressure and does not correct the renal or systemic activity of the RAAS. These differences in baseline characteristics (blood pressure and renin activity) may indicate that this population was younger, had lower baseline RAS activation, potentially explaining differences between the studies. The 8-week duration of treatment may have been inadequate to affect RAS activity or blood pressure. Although the researchers were able to restore plasma vitamin D levels to normal in the treatment group within 8 weeks, it is assumed that a longer treatment period would be required for the full effect of vitamin D on blood pressure and on RAAS activity.

It is known that increased central or renal sympathetic activation is an important factor in the pathogenesis of human arterial hypertension. There is still no evidence that vitamin D deficiency directly affects sympathetic nervous activity. It is assumed that vitamin D deficiency enhances the signaling effect caused by increased sympathetic activity. For example, angiotensin II promotes hypertension due to increased activation of T cells in the central nervous system, and vitamin D blocks the activity of effector T cells. In this way, vitamin D deficiency enhances the sympathetic effect stimulated by the T cells [30].

The relationship between the development of CVD and low levels of 25-hydroxy-vitamin D in individuals initially without cardiovascular disease was also identified in the prospective study, The Framingham Offspring Study. In this study, with an average duration of 5.4 years, 1739 participants were observed, the average concentration of 25-OH D was 19.7 ng/ml (25-OH D ˂ 15 ng/ml-9%), and the results showed that different kinds of CVDs developed more often in persons with vitamin D deficiency [31].

Studies conducted in Germany for 7.7 years in which 3258 patients with CVD over 20 years old were observed proves that the risk of death from CVD increases two times in those patients whose vitamin D level is below normal, as well as an increase in the level of C-reactive protein and interleukin-6 is also observed in patients with low levels of vitamin D [32, 33]. These and other studies confirm that blood pressure and C-reactive protein levels are inversely related to vitamin D in blood serum. The authors found gender differences in the prevalence of hypertension depending on vitamin D levels. The researchers found hypertension in 50% of women who had very low vitamin D levels (<5 ng/ml) compared with 30% of women who had vitamin D levels not less than 20 ng/ml. No differences in the prevalence of arterial hypertension depending on the level of vitamin D were found among men. Among 4863 participants in the Women's Health Initiative study, over 7 years of follow-up, there was no association between vitamin D levels and changes in blood pressure [34]. But women with plasma vitamin D levels <14 ng/ml had a 50% increased risk of arterial hypertension compared with women with higher vitamin D levels (19–26 ng/ml). In a Michigan study, 413 women with an average vitamin D level of 24 ± 10 ng/ml had higher diastolic blood pressure values (77 ± 9 mm Hg) compared with women with normal vitamin D levels—vitamin D ≥ 32 ng/ml; 75 ± 9 mm Hg [35]. Cross-sectional study with 833 white men who underwent 24-hour blood pressure monitoring (excellent outcome assessment) found that low vitamin D levels (<15 ng/mL) are associated with higher prevalence of hypertension [36].

5. Vitamin D in elderly patients

It was reported that in elderly patients with systolic hypertension, supplementation with vitamin D deficiency did not significantly affect blood pressure. In 2013, Witham et al. [37] reported the VitDISH study results. The study enrolled 159 participants with a mean age of 77 years, mean BP of 163/78 mmHg, and an average level of 25 (OH) D of 18 ng/ml. Participants received 100,000 IU of oral vitamin D3 or a placebo every 3 months for 1 year. Treatment increased 25 (OH) D levels by 8 ng/ml, but did not show significant reductions in blood pressure and arterial stiffness in selected patients with systolic hypertension, which was apparently associated with increased vascular stiffness and calcification. Although these patients were taking one to two antihypertensive drugs, their systolic blood pressure was about 160 mm Hg [37]. In another study on the effect of vitamin D on blood pressure in elderly patients with systolic hypertension, people aged 75 years were treated with (mean BP 144/85 mm Hg, 25 (OH) D 10.1 ng/ml, n = 74) 800 IU vitamin D plus 1200 mg calcium daily for eight weeks. They found a significant increase in 25 (OH) D levels and a decrease in systolic blood pressure with vitamin D and calcium supplementation compared with calcium alone. Clearly, well-designed placebo-controlled trials using 2000–3000 IU of vitamin D daily to treat patients with isolated systolic hypertension and vitamin D deficiency are warranted [38]. The BEST-D study in healthy people examined the effect of daily vitamin D intake for 1 year on the risk of hypertension and biochemical markers. But the results of this study were not positive. The addition of vitamin D did increase the plasma concentration of 25 (OH), but did not reduce the risk of cardiovascular complications, blood pressure, blood lipid profile, and arterial stiffness [39].

6. Clinical trials with vitamin D in hypertension

More than 40 randomized clinical trials have been conducted to determine the effect of vitamin D supplementation on blood pressure as a primary or secondary endpoint. Since the mechanisms underlying the effect of vitamin D on blood pressure have not yet been elucidated, most clinical trials have shown suboptimal designs, and the results have been mixed. The findings were conflicting. Wu et al. [40] conducted a meta-analysis of four randomized controlled trials of oral vitamin D supplementation in BP. They found that vitamin D supplementation significantly reduced systolic blood pressure by 2.44 mm Hg, but not diastolic blood pressure. Another meta-analysis included 51 randomized trials that enrolled adults who received vitamin D supplementation and that measured several cardiovascular outcomes (stroke, myocardial infarction, cardiovascular death, etc.) [41] found no change in the weighted mean of either systolic or diastolic blood pressure.

Witham et al. [42] investigated eight randomized controlled trials in participants with a mean baseline blood pressure > 140/90 mm Hg, which showed a slight decrease in systolic blood pressure and a small significant decrease in diastolic blood pressure (3.1 mm Hg). In a study involving 701 adolescent girls and boys with average blood vitamin D values of 30 ng/ml, it was shown that there is an inverse correlation between the level of this vitamin and the values of systolic and diastolic blood pressure (respectively, $r = -0.1$, $r = -0.21$; $P < 0.01$) [43]. In a subanalysis of the Hoorn population study in the Netherlands, which included 441 patients, it was shown that blood pressure levels decreased with increasing blood vitamin D values. With the values of vitamin D in plasma on average 32 ng/ml, the systolic and diastolic pressures were respectively 135.0 ± 18.6 mm Hg and 81.6 ± 9.6 mm Hg. At low values of vitamin D in the blood, below 14 ng/ml, the values of systolic and diastolic pressure were 146.6 ± 20.6 mm Hg and 86.3 ± 12.6 mm Hg [44].

Ten studies by other scientists examined the role of vitamin D and ultraviolet radiation in blood pressure regulation, where no significant effect of vitamin D on blood pressure was found. Only those studies using high daily doses of vitamin D (at least 1000 IU/day) were found to have a small statistically significant effect [45]. An ideal test to determine the maximum antihypertensive effect of vitamin D supplementation on blood pressure is the administration of vitamin D to patients with untreated stage 1 hypertension with vitamin D deficiency living in high latitudes in winter. Such a study was conducted ($n = 40$) in Liaoning, northern China, in the winter, administering 3000 IU of vitamin D daily for 3 weeks to patients with an average age of 53 years who did not receive treatment for stage 1 EH and vitamin D deficiency (25 (OH) D levels were < 20 ng/ml). Treatment significantly increased blood 25 (OH) D levels and decreased systolic blood pressure, but not diastolic blood pressure. The negative results for diastolic blood pressure may be associated with a small sample size, a short treatment period, and a recruitment of only stage 1 hypertensive patients. A well-designed, large, randomized study VITAL has demonstrated a significant reduction in the incidence of hypertension after 5 years of vitamin D intake (2000 IU per day) by eliminating vitamin D deficiency in patients aged ≥50 years [46]. It should be noted that an appropriately high dose (at least>1000 IU per day) of vitamin D supplementation to increase blood 25 (OH) D levels is also needed to see the antihypertensive effect of vitamin D.

Kunutsor et al. [47] conducted a meta-analysis of 16 randomized clinical trials to evaluate the effect of vitamin D supplementation on blood pressure. They did not show significant reductions in systolic and diastolic blood pressure with vitamin D supplementation, suggesting heterogeneity and publication bias. Subgroup analysis showed significant reductions in diastolic blood pressure in participants with preexisting cardiometabolic disease.

The VITAL trial did not find any significant benefits in regard to cardiovascular outcomes. Indeed, only a not significant reduction in cardiovascular events was observed in the group treated with vitamin D when compared with the placebo [48]. In other studies, cholecalciferol supplementation did not reduce the cardiovascular risk. This treatment increased the serum levels of 25(OH)D, the CVD risk did not improve [49]. Another meta-analysis evaluated the cardiovascular benefits of a vitamin D supplementation over 1 year, regardless of calcium supplementation. The results of this meta-analysis showed no significant effect of vitamin D on cardiovascular endpoints (myocardial infarction, cerebral stroke, cerebrovascular accident, mortality from heart disease) and on mortality from all causes [50].

It should be noted that the development of acute toxic effects during treatment with vitamin D is very rare, since the toxicity of this vitamin can be caused by the use of very high doses. Such toxic effects may include hypercalcemia, which stimulates the development of various types of arrhythmias with a shortened QT interval [51]. No less controversial is the issue of vitamin D toxicity. So, according to I. Boer et al. [52], safe level of 25 (OH) D3 in plasma is considered to be 240 nmol/l, the concentration of 25 (OH) D3 in the blood is higher, 375 nmol/L, associated with acute hypercalcemia and hyperphosphatemia. With that said, American Institute of Medicine determines the maximum daily intake of vitamin D for infants from 0 up to 6 months of life 1000 IU; for children from 7 to 12 months life—1500 IU; from 1 to 3 years—2500 IU; from 4 up to 8 years—3000 IU; for teenagers from 9 to 18 years old and adults—4000 IU.

There are small studies in the literature that investigated the effect of vitamin D on blood pressure when taken daily at a dose of 3000 IU versus placebo [53]. As a result of these studies, taking vitamin D did not lead to a significant decrease in blood pressure. However, in a retrospective analysis, patients with vitamin D deficiency (<32 ng/ml) showed a decrease in systolic and diastolic blood pressure during treatment with vitamin D. However, the central systolic blood pressure (blood pressure in the ascending aorta) decreased by 4 mm Hg in the 25(OH)D group compared with placebo ($P = 0.007$). The results of these studies confirm that the addition of vitamin D to the treatment of hypertensive patients may be beneficial in patients with vitamin D deficiency. It should be noted that high doses of vitamin D were used. In addition, patients with systolic blood pressure levels <150 or diastolic blood pressure < 95 mm Hg, and 84% of participants were taking antihypertensive drugs. All this could mask or reduce the effect of vitamin D on blood pressure in hypertensive patients. These factors, along with the small sample size, may have contributed significantly to negative 24-hour BP outcomes. Besides, most studies did not record the changes of diet, sun exposure or latitudes, genetic factors, and educational status, we are not able to answer the questions of whether these factors would modify the effect of the intervention.

A meta-analysis of cohort studies was conducted that demonstrated a negative association between vitamin D levels and blood pressure. At the same time, with an increase in the level of vitamin D in blood plasma by 25 nmol/l, a decrease in the risk of developing arterial hypertension by 7% was observed. However, there was no direct evidence of a decrease in blood pressure from 25 (OH) D supplementation. Scientists believe that the positive effect of vitamin D on blood pressure levels is mainly due to the fact that the study included young participants with a healthy lifestyle. In addition, low vitamin D levels may be the result of prior medical conditions. Furthermore, differences exist among the various methods used and in the laboratories that measured 25(OH)D levels, which would also influence the accuracy of the study results. Individuals who are taking vitamin D supplements should do so for at least 6 months to reach the maximum attained 25(OH)D level. It is reasonable to assume that the effect of vitamin D is time-dependent [54].

Beveridge et al. [55] conducted a meta-analysis that included clinical trials that used vitamin D supplements and reported BP. Vitamin D did not affect normal blood pressure in 30 studies. They also found no significant reduction in blood pressure with vitamin D in studies with participants whose mean baseline SBP was ≥140 mmHg. The main reason for negative results may be related to suboptimal study design. This may include high rates of background antihypertensive drug treatment that overlap with the antihypertensive role of vitamin D, cohorts with less than 40% of participants with vitamin D deficiency, and low or exceptionally high intake of vitamin D. Chen et al. [56] conducted a placebo-controlled, randomized study to find out if vitamin D supplementation (2000 IU/day) lowered blood pressure for 6 months. The study included 126 patients with arterial hypertension and vitamin D deficiency who received nifedipine at a dose of 30 mg per day. For 6 months of treatment with vitamin D, an increase in its level was observed from 19 ng/ml to 34 ng/ml and a decrease in mean blood pressure over 24 hours by 6.2/4.2 mm Hg. ($p < 0.001$). In patients with vitamin D < 30 ng/ml at baseline ($n = 113$), the mean blood pressure in 24 hours decreased by 7.1/5.7 mm Hg. In this study, the antihypertensive drug nifedipine could reduce the effects of vitamin D on blood pressure in these Chinese hypertensive patients.

7. Vitamin D, endothelial dysfunction, and atherosclerosis

The endothelium is the main regulator of vascular homeostasis and affects vasoconstriction and vasodilation, smooth muscle proliferation and inflammation, thrombogenesis, and fibrinolysis. As a result, the development of atherosclerosis occurs with endothelial dysfunction, which develops when this layer of the vascular wall is damaged. The role of vitamin D in reducing the risk of atherosclerosis lies in the following mechanisms:

- increase in the formation of endothelial nitric oxide
- decrease in aggregation and adhesion of platelets
- management of musculoskeletal tone
- suppression of oxidative stress
- decrease in the formation of pro-inflammatory cytokines

- decrease in the formation of vasoconstrictor substances
- inhibition of proliferation and migration of smooth muscle cells
- modulation of the immune response.

Vitamin D has beneficial effects on vascular endothelial function and arterial stiffness. Vitamin D plays an important role in vascular and endothelial smooth muscle cells. Therefore, it can be assumed that vitamin D can affect the contraction of blood vessels and the formation of calcifications in the vessels. At the same time, this vitamin can affect the function and structure of blood vessels in different ways. Everyone knows that nitric oxide is a powerful vasoprotective and vasodilator, and several factors are involved in its synthesis, including vitamin D and vitamin D receptors. Scientists believe that vitamin D plays an essential role in the synthesis of nitric oxide. Other mechanisms include endothelial 1-hydroxylase and activated vitamin D, which can modulate the growth of both cell types [3]. In patients with type 2 diabetes, the DIMENSION study examined the effect of 16 weeks of vitamin D supplementation on endothelial function. During the treatment, the values of vitamin D increased. But when conducting a multivariate regression analysis, no effects of vitamin D on endothelial function were found [57].

Arterial stiffness increases in early-stage hypertensive patients, and it is a strong predictor of cardiovascular morbidity and mortality. In a study, Sinem Cakal [23] included 100 patients with arterial hypertension who were diagnosed for the first time, they had not previously received antihypertensive treatment, they did not have any cardiovascular diseases, chronic renal pathology, diabetes mellitus, malignant neoplasms. All patients were divided into two groups: with vitamin D deficiency (<20 ng/ml) and with normal vitamin D content (≥20 ng/ml). The daytime, nighttime, and daily blood pressures were determined. In the result, vitamin D deficiency is associated with increased arterial stiffness in newly diagnosed hypertensive patients.

Everyone knows that inflammation plays an important role in the development of atherosclerosis. The most widely studied biomarker of cardiovascular inflammation with proven anti-inflammatory effects is highly sensitive C-reactive protein. Many studies have shown an inverse relationship between vitamin D and reactive protein C [58, 59]. The level of vitamin D is positively correlated with the concentration of anti-inflammatory cytokines (interleukin 10), which enhances the anti-inflammatory effect of vitamin D. By reducing the production of pro-inflammatory cytokines, interleukin 10 has a cardioprotective effect. A decrease in the level of this interleukin in the blood leads to the development of severe atherosclerosis. Thanks to this mechanism, vitamin D is able to slow down the progress of atherosclerosis. In addition, vitamin D is able to suppress the formation of pro-inflammatory tumor necrosis factor, which once again proves the indisputable role of this vitamin in the development of inflammation. With vitamin D deficiency in the body, the synthesis of atherogenic cholesterol fractions increases, which leads to an increase in atherosclerotic processes in the body. The effect of vitamin D is comparable to the effect of statins, since it inhibits the enzyme HMG-CoA reductase—3-hydroxy-3-methylglutaryl-coenzyme A-reductase, which is an important link in the pathogenesis of atherosclerosis [60].

Several findings currently suggest that there is a link between the vitamin D system and the development of atherosclerotic plaques, possibly mediated by a modulation of immune responses [61]. This study showed that in patients with diabetes mellitus, vitamin D can affect signaling from vitamin D receptors on the surface of macrophages, which leads to a decrease in the penetration of LDL cholesterol into foam cells, which prevents the development of atherosclerosis. Due to the inhibition of the nuclear factor of gene expression of activated B cells, vitamin D suppresses the synthesis of prothrombogenic and pro-inflammatory cytokines (interleukin 6) and also increases the formation of anti-inflammatory interleukin 10 and thrombomodulin. All this leads to a decrease in vascular calcification and stops the development of atherosclerotic plaques by suppressing the formation of foam cells.

W. John et al. [62] when carrying out an analysis using multivariate models, including the fact the risk of developing diabetes mellitus and ischemic heart disease, found that vitamin D deficiency helps to reduce the content of apolipoprotein A1. Another study carried out with the aim elucidating the relationship between vitamin D content and metabolic risk factors in young men rank without obesity proved that the content in the blood circulator 25 (OH) D3 correlated with the level of LDL [63]. Results of a randomized trial, conducted by G. Major, et al. [64], testimony about the fact that the daily intake of 400 IU of cholecalciferol and 1200 mg calcium led to a decrease total cholesterol levels.

8. The place of vitamin D in the development of chronic heart failure

For the first time in 1995, L. Brunvand et al. [65] presented a clinical case of the association of pronounced vitamin D deficiency, hypocalcemia with myocardial dysfunction, and chronic heart failure. E. Shane et al. [66] proved statistically significant predominance of vitamin D deficiency in patients with chronic heart failure, direct correlation between the level of vitamin D it contains in serum and a fraction of left ventricular throw. A. Zittermann et al. [67] demonstrated low serum 25 (OH) D3 and calcitriol levels in the blood of patients with chronic heart failure sufficiency in comparison with the control group healthy people. The authors have proven that the connection between vitamin D deficiency and chronic heart failure sufficiency is traced in all age groups, with the correlation of the relationship between the low level of 25 (OH) D3 and an increased content of cerebral sodium uretic peptide. Prospective cross-examination and follow-up performed by A. Zittermann et al. demonstrated statistically significant prevalence of vitamin D deficiency in patients with indications for emergency heart transplantation in comparison with patients preparing for a planned transplantation. A lower circulating level vitamin D has been associated with a risk of sudden heart death. Research results of I. Gotsman et al. [68] testified to a statistically significant possessing a deficiency of 25 (OH) D3 in patients with chronic heart failure in comparison with control. The authors proved that less than 9% of such patients had an optimal level of 25 (OH) D3, highlighting significantly adverse consequences of its deficiency. Thus, the carried out studies show that there is a statistically significant prevalence of vitamin D deficiency in patients with chronic heart failure in comparison with nursing patients without it; vitamin D deficiency is associated with the severity of heart failure and higher rates of unfavorable outcomes.

In 2016, a 26.5-month study was completed to establish the incidence of vitamin D deficiency and its relationship with bone mineral density, left ventricular ejection fraction, and brain natriuretic peptide (NT-proBNP) levels. Two groups were formed: the first included 70 patients with chronic heart failure (CHF); the second—40 patients with diseases of the cardiovascular system, but without CHF. Osteoporosis was detected in 61.4% of patients in the first group (they had fractures much more often) and in

32.5% of patients in the second group. In patients with CHF, a statistically significant decrease in the level of vitamin D was recorded, on average, this value was 9.6 ng/ml, in patients without CHF—14.8 ng/ml, and in patients of group 1, a high level of NT-proBNP was observed. A correlation was found between the level of vitamin D in serum and the concentration of NT-proBNP, the left ventricular ejection fraction. As a result, it was concluded that patients with CHF are a group at increased risk of osteoporosis, and such patients are recommended to prescribe additional vitamin D intake at a dosage of more than 1600 IU per day as a preventive measure [69]. The pathophysiological mechanisms of these relationships are not fully understood, there are various hypotheses, according to one—vitamin D deficiency contributes to the development of secondary hyperparathyroidism. A high level of parathyroid hormone provokes calcification of the heart valves (this is especially pronounced in patients with renal failure), as a result of which the risk of developing CHF increases. The reason for the development of CHF is also the "aging" of the myocardium; the key factors that determine the rate of aging are oxidative stress and chronic inflammation. Vitamin D deficiency is associated with a higher incidence of heart failure due to an increase in serum pro-inflammatory markers, including CRP [52, 53, 70].

9. Conclusion

Based on the evidence presented, it can be assumed that the correction of the deficit of vitamin D will help reduce the risk occurrence and progression of cardiovascular diseases, reducing the risk of sudden cardiac death and general mortality of the population.

Based on the conducted studies, it is assumed that the risk of developing arterial hypertension can be explained by the initial content of vitamin D in the blood, sample size, and duration of observation. In addition, the presence of other concomitant cardiovascular diseases, diabetes mellitus, kidney disease, affects the physiological mechanisms of the effect of vitamin D on blood pressure. Therefore, between individual patients there may be significant differences in the physiological effects of vitamin D.

Thus, arterial hypertension is caused by a variety of factors acting through genetic and environmental determinants depending on age. Vitamin D deficiency as a risk factor for the environment contributes to an increase in vascular tone, which, possibly, serves as a trigger that contributes to the development of hypertension in vulnerable middle-aged people. Accumulating data from animal models and observational studies in humans strongly support the hypothesis that vitamin D deficiency contributes to hypertension, and a corresponding high dose of vitamin D with long-term treatment can normalize or nearly normalize blood 25 (OH) D levels and significantly reduce blood pressure in groups of hypertensive patients with vitamin D deficiency.

Correction of vitamin D deficiency is of great prognostic value. Vitamin D treatment is low-cost, easy to administer, and prevention further contributes to a healthy lifestyle. Further clinical and experimental studies are needed to study in more detail the mechanisms of the negative effect of vitamin D deficiency on the cardiovascular system, in particular on arterial hypertension.

Author details

Sona Gahramanova
Clinical Pharmacology Department, Azerbaijan Medical University, Baku, Azerbaijan

*Address all correspondence to: sonaxanum@mail.ru

References

[1] Parati G, Stergiou G, O'Brien E, Asmar R, Beilin L, Bilo G, et al. European Society of Hypertension practice guidelines for ambulatory blood pressure monitoring. Journal of Hypertension. 2014;**32**(7):1359-1366

[2] Pilz S, Gaksch M, Kienreich K, Grubler M, Verheyen N, Fahrleitner-Pammer A, et al. Effects of vitamin D on blood pressure and cardiovascular risk factors: A randomized controlled trial. Hypertension. 2015;**65**(6):1195-1201

[3] Legarth C, Grimm D, Wehland M, Bauer J, Krüger M. The Impact of Vitamin D in the Treatment of Essential Hypertension. International Journal of Molecular Sciences. 2018;**19**:455

[4] Holick MF. Vitamin D deficiency. The New England Journal of Medicine. 2007;**357**(3):266-281

[5] Martins D, Wolf M, Pan D, et al. Prevalence of cardiovascular risk factors and the serumlevels of 25-hydroxyvitamin D in the United States: Data from the Third National Health and Nutrition Examination Survey. Archives of Internal Medicine. 2007;**167**(11):1159-1165

[6] Bouillon R, Carmeliet G, Verlinden L, van Etten E, Verstuyf A, Luderer HF, et al. Vitamin D and human health: Lessons from vitamin D receptor null mice. Endocrine Reviews. 2008;**29**(6):726-776

[7] Xiang W, Kong J, Chen S, Cao LP, Qiao G, Zheng W, et al. Cardiac hypertrophy in vitamin D receptor knockout mice: Role of the systemic and cardiac renin-angiotensin systems. American Journal of Physiology Endocrinology and Metabolism. 2005;**288**(1):E125-E132

[8] Mozaffari-Khosravi H, Loloei S, Mirjalili MR, Barzegar K. The effect of vitamin D supplementation on blood pressure in patients with elevated blood pressure and vitamin D deficiency: A randomized, double-blind, placebo-controlled trial. Blood Pressure Monitoring. 2015;**20**(2):83-91

[9] Magurno M, Crescibene D, Spinali M, Cassano V, Armentaro G, Barbara K, et al. Vitamin D and subclinical cardiovascular damage in essential hypertension. Endocrine. 2021;**2**:13

[10] Institute of Medicine Food and Nutrition Board. Dietary reference intakes for calcium and vitamin D. Washington (DC): The National Academies Press; 2011

[11] Wong MSK, Delansorne R, Man RYK, et al. Chronic treatment with vitamin D lowers arterial blood pressure and reduces endothelium-dependent contractions in the aorta of the spontaneously hypertensive rat. American Journal of Physiology. Heart and Circulatory Physiology. 2010;**299**(4):H1226-H1234

[12] Lind L, Lithell H, Skarfors E, Wide L, Ljunghall S. Reduction of blood pressure by treatment with alphacalcidol. A double-blind, placebo-controlled study in subjects with impaired glucose tolerance. Acta Medica Scandinavica. 1988;**223**:211-217

[13] Rostand SG. Vitamin D, blood pressure, and African Americans: Toward a unifying hypothesis. Clinical Journal of the American Society of Nephrology: CJASN. 2010;**5**:1697-1703

[14] Krause R, Buhring M, Hopfenmuller W, Holick MF,

Sharma AM. Ultraviolet B and blood pressure. Lancet. 1998;**352**:709-710

[15] Liu X, Baylin A, PD L. Vitamin D deficiency and insufficiency among US adults: Prevalence, predictors and clinical implications. The British Journal of Nutrition. 2018;**119**(8):928-936. DOI: 10.1017/S0007114518000491

[16] Romero DC, Manson J. Vitamin D and your heart. Circulation. 2015;**132**(25):391-392

[17] Vimaleswaran KS, Cavadino A, Berry DJ, Jorde R, Dieffenbach AK, Lu C, et al. Association of vitamin D status with arterial blood pressure and hypertension risk: A mendelian randomisation study. The Lancet Diabetes and Endocrinology. 2014; **2**(9):719-729

[18] Burgaz A, Orsini N, Larsson SC, Wolk A. Blood 25-hydroxyvitamin D concentration and hypertension: A meta-analysis. Journal of Hypertension. 2011;**29**:636-645

[19] Forman JP, Scott JB, Ng K, Drake BF, Suarez EG, Hayden DL, et al. Effect of vitamin D supplementation on blood pressure in blacks. Hypertension. 2013;**61**:779-785

[20] Kunutsor SK, Apekey TA, Steur M. Vitamin D and risk of future hypertension: Meta-analysis of 283,537 participants. European Journal of Epidemiology. 2013;**28**(3):205-221

[21] Li YC, Kong J, Wei M, Chen ZF, Liu SQ, Cao LP. 1,25-Dihydroxyvitamin D(3) is a negative endocrine regulator of the renin-angiotensin system. The Journal of Clinical Investigation. 2002;**110**(2):229-238

[22] Chen S, Sun Y, Agrawal DK. Vitamin D deficiency and essential hypertension. Journal of the American Society of Hypertension. 2015;**9**(11):885-901

[23] Cakal S, Çakal B, Karaca O. Association of vitamin D deficiency with arterial stiffness in newly diagnosed hypertension. Blood Pressure Monitoring. 2021;**26**(2):113-117. DOI: 10.1097/MBP.0000000000000497

[24] Zhou C, Lu F, Cao K, Xu D, Goltzman D, Miao D. Calcium-independent and 1,25(OH)2D3-dependent regulation of the renin-angiotensin system in 1alpha-hydroxylase knockout mice. Kidney International. 2008;**74**(2):170-179

[25] Beierwaltes WH. The role of calcium in the regulation of renin secretion. American Journal of Physiology Renal Physiology. 2010;**298**(1):F1-F11

[26] Vaidya A, Forman JP, Williams JS. Vitamin D and the vascular sensitivity to angiotensin II in obese caucasians with hypertension. Journal of Human Hypertension. 2011;**25**(11):672-678

[27] Vaidya A, Sun B, Forman JP, Hopkins PN, Brown NJ, Kolatkar NS, et al. The Fok1 vitamin D receptor gene polymorphism is associated with plasma renin activity in Caucasians. Clinical Endocrinology. 2011;**74**(6):783-790

[28] Vaidya A, Sun B, Larson C, Forman JP, Williams JS. Vitamin D3 therapy corrects the tissue sensitivity to angiotensin ii akin to the action of a converting enzyme inhibitor in obese hypertensives: An interventional study. The Journal of Clinical Endocrinology and Metabolism. 2012;**97**(7):2456-2465

[29] McMullan CJ, Borgi L, Curhan GC, Fisher N, Forman JP. The effect of vitamin D on renin-angiotensin-system activation and blood pressure—A randomized control trial. Journal of

Hypertension. 2017;**35**(4):822-829. DOI: 10.1097/HJH.0000000000001220

[30] Guzik TJ, Hoch NE, Brown KA, McCann LA, Rahman A, Dikalov S, et al. Role of the T cell in the genesis of angiotensin II induced hypertension and vascular dysfunction. The Journal of Experimental Medicine. 2007;**204**:2449-2460

[31] Wang TJ et al. Vitamin D deficiency and risk of cardiovascular disease. Circulation. 2008;**117**(4):503-511. DOI: 10.1161/CIRCULATIONAHA. 107.706127

[32] Dobnig H, Pilz S, Scharnage H, et al. Independent association of low serum 25-hudroxyvitamin D and 1,25-Di-hydroxyvitamin D levels with all-cause and cardio-vascular mortality. Archives of Internal Medicine. 2008;**168**(12):1340-1349. DOI: 10.1001/archinte.168.12.1340

[33] Hintzpeter B, Mensink GBM, Thierfelder W, et al. Vitamin D status and health correlates among German adults. European Journal of Clinical Nutrition. 2008;**62**(9):1079-1089

[34] Margolis KL, Martin LW, Ray RM, et al. A prospective study of serum 25-hydroxyvitamin D levels, blood pressure, and incident hypertension in postmenopausal women. American Journal of Epidemiology. 2012;**175**(1):22-32

[35] Griffin FC, Gadegbeku CA, Sowers MR. Vitamin D and subsequent systolic hypertension among women. American Journal of Hypertension. 2011;**24**(3):316-321

[36] Burgaz A, Byberg L, Rautiainen S, et al. Confirmed hypertension and plasma 25(OH)D concentrations amongst elderly men. Journal of Internal Medicine. 2011;**269**(2):211-218

[37] Witham MD, Price RJ, Struthers AD, Donnan PT, Messow CM, Ford I, et al. Cholecalciferol treatment to reduce blood pressure in older patients with isolated systolic hypertension: The VitDISH randomized controlled trial. JAMA Internal Medicine. 2013;**173**:1672-1679

[38] Pfeifer M, Begerow B, Minne HW, Nachtigall D, Hansen C. Effects of a short-term vitamin D(3) and calcium supplementation on blood pressure and parathyroid hormone levels in elderly women. The Journal of Clinical Endocrinology and Metabolism. 2001;**86**:1633-1637

[39] Hin H, Tomson J, Newman C, Kurien R, Lay M, Cox J, et al. Optimum dose of vitamin D for disease prevention in older people: BEST-D trial of vitamin D in primary care. Osteoporosis International. 2017;**28**:841-851

[40] Wu SH, Ho SC, Zhong L. Effects of vitamin D supplementation on blood pressure. Southern Medical Journal. 2010;**103**:729-737

[41] Elamin MB, Abu Elnour NO, Elamin KB, et al. Vitamin D and cardiovascular outcomes: A systematic review and meta-analysis. The Journal of Clinical Endocrinology and Metabolism. 2011;**96**(7):1931-1942

[42] Witham MD, Nadir MA, Struthers AD. Effect of vitamin D on blood pressure: A systematic review and meta-analysis. Journal of Hypertension. 2009;**27**:1948-1954

[43] Parikh S, Guo D-H, Pollock NK, et al. Circulating 25-hydroxyvitamin D concentrations are correlated with cardiometabolic risk among American black and white adolescents living in a year-round sunny climate. Diabetes Care. 2012;**35**(5):1133-1138

[44] van Ballegooijen AJ, Snijder MB, Visser M, et al. Vitamin D in relation to myocardial structure and function after eight years of follow-up: The Hoorn study. Annals of Nutrition & Metabolism. 2012;**60**(1):69-77

[45] Pittas AG, Chung M, Trikalinos T, Mitri J, Brendel M, Patel K, et al. Systematic review: Vitamin D and cardiometabolic outcomes. Annals of Internal Medicine. 2010;**152**:307-314

[46] Manson JE, Bassuk SS, Lee IM, Cook NR, Albert MA, Gordon D, et al. The VITamin D and OmegA-3 TriaL (VITAL): Rationale and design of a large randomized controlled trial of vitamin D and marine omega-3 fatty acid supplements for the primary prevention of cancer and cardiovascular disease. Contemporary Clinical Trials. 2012;**33**:159-171

[47] Kunutsor SK, Burgess S, Munroe PB, Khan H. Vitamin D and high blood pressure: Causal association or epiphenomenon? European Journal of Epidemiology. 2014;**29**:1-14

[48] Manson JE, Cook NR, Lee IM, Christen W, Bassuk SS, Mora S, et al. Vitamin D supplements and prevention of cancer and cardiovascular disease. The New England Journal of Medicine. 2019;**380**:33-44

[49] Legarth C, Grimm D, Krüger M, Infanger M, Wehland M. Potential beneficial effects of vitamin D in coronary artery disease. Nutrients. 2019;**12**:99

[50] Barbarawi M, Kheiri B, Zayed Y, Barbarawi O, Dhillon H, Swaid B, et al. Vitamin D supplementation and cardiovascular disease risks in more than 83,000 individuals in 21 randomized clinical trials: A meta-analysis. JAMA Cardiology. 2019;**4**:765-776

[51] De la Guía-Galipienso F, Martínez-Ferran M, Vallecillo N, Lavie CJ, Sanchis-Gomar F, Pareja-Galeano H. Vitamin D and cardiovascular health. Clinical Nutrition. 2021;**40**:2946-2957

[52] Boer IH, Kestenbaum B, Shoben AB, Michos ED, Sarnak MJ, Siscovick DS. 25-Hydroxyvitamin D levels inversely associate with risk for developing coronary artery calcification. Journal of the American Society of Nephrology. 2009;**20**:1805-1812. DOI: 10.1681/ASN.2008111157

[53] Larsen T, Mose FH, Bech JN, et al. Effect of cholecalciferol supplementation during winter months in patients with hypertension: A randomized, placebo-controlled trial. American Journal of Hypertension. 2012;**25**(11):1215-1222

[54] Zhang D, Cheng C, Wang Y, et al. Effect of vitamin D on blood pressure and hypertension in the general population: An update meta-analysis of cohort studies and randomized controlled trials. Preventing Chronic Disease. 2020;**17**:E03. DOI: 10.5888/pcd17.190307

[55] Beveridge LA, Struthers AD, Khan F, Jorde R, Scragg R, Macdonald HM, et al. Effect of vitamin D supplementation on blood pressure: A systematic review and meta-analysis incorporating individual patient data. JAMA Internal Medicine. 2015;**175**(5):745-754

[56] Chen WR, Liu ZY, Shi Y, Yin da W, Wang H, Sha Y, et al. Vitamin D and nifedipine in the treatment of Chinese patients with grades I-II essential hypertension: A randomized placebo-controlled trial. Atherosclerosis. 2014;**235**:102-109

[57] Dalan R, Liew H, Assam PN, Chan ES, Siddiqui FJ, Tan AW, et al. A randomized controlled trial evaluating the impact of targeted vitamin D

supplementation on endothelial function in type 2 diabetes mellitus: The dimension trial. Diabetes and Vascular Disease Research. 2016;**13**:192-200

[58] Carlson N, Mah R, Aburto M, Peters MJ, Dupper MV, Chen LH. Hypovitaminosis D. Correction and high-sensitivity C-reactive protein levels in hypertensive adults. The Permanente Journal. 2013;**17**(4):19-21. DOI: 10.7812/tpp/13-007

[59] Liefaard MC, Ligthart S, Vitezova A, Hofman A, Uitterlinden AG, Kiefte-de Jong JC, et al. Vitamin D and C-reactive protein: A mendelian randomization study. PLoS One. 2015;**10**(7):e0131740. DOI: 10.1371/journal.pone.0131740

[60] Kane L, Moore K, Lütjohann D, et al. Vitamin D3 effects on lipids differ in statin and nonstatin-treated humans: Superiority of free 25-OH D levels in detecting relationships. The Journal of Clinical Endocrinology and Metabolism. 2013;**98**(11):4400-4409. DOI: 10.1210/jc.2013-1922

[61] Oh J, Weng S, Felton SK, Bhandare S, Riek A, Butler B, et al. 1,25(OH)2 vitamin d inhibits foam cell formation and suppresses macrophage cholesterol uptake in patients with type 2 diabetes mellitus. Circulation. 2009;**120**:687-698

[62] John WG, Noonan K, Mannan N, Boucher BJ. Hypovitaminosis D is associated with reductions in serum apolipoprotein A-I but not with fasting lipids in British Bangladeshis. The American Journal of Clinical Nutrition. 2005;**82**:517-522. DOI: 10.1093/ajcn.82.3.517

[63] Gannage-Yared M, Chedid R, Khalife S, Azzi E, Zoghbi F, Halaby G. Vitamin D in relation to metabolic risk factors, insulin sensitivity and adiponectin in a young middle eastern population. European Journal of Endocrinology. 2009;**160**:965-971. DOI: 10.1530/EJE-08-0952

[64] Major GC, Alarie F, Dore J. Supplementation with calcium+vitamin D enhances the beneficial effect of weight loss on plasma lipid and lipoprotein concentrations. The American Journal of Clinical Nutrition. 2007;**85**:54-59. DOI: 10.1093/ajcn/85.1.54

[65] Brunvand L, Haga P, Tangsrud SE, Haug E. Congestive heart failure caused by vitamin D deficiency? Acta Paediatrica. 1995;**84**:106-108

[66] Shane E, Mancini D, Aaronson K. Bone mass, vitamin D deficiency, and hyperparathyroidism in congestive heart failure. The American Journal of Medicine. 1997;**103**:197-207

[67] Zittermann A, Schleithoff SS, Tenderich G. Low vitamin D status: A contributing factor in the pathogenesis of congestive heart failure? Journal of the American College of Cardiology. 2003;**41**:105-112

[68] Gotsman I, Shauer A, Zwas DR, Hellman Y, Keren A, Lotan C, et al. Vitamin D deficiency is a predictor of reduced survival in patients with heart failure; vitamin D supplementation improves outcome. European Journal of Heart Failure. 2012;**14**:357-366. DOI: 10.1093/eurjhf/hfr175

[69] Larina VN, Raspopova TN. Mineral bone density and bone metabolism in chronic heart failure. Kardiologiia. 2016;**56**(7):33-45. DOI: 10.18565/cardio.2016.7.39-46

[70] Judd SE, Raiser SN, Kumari M, Tangpricha V. 1,25-dihydroxyvitamin D3 reduces systolic blood pressure in hypertensive adults: A pilot feasibility study. The Journal of Steroid Biochemistry and Molecular Biology. 2010;**121**(1-2):445-447

Chapter 5

Self-Management Strategies in Outpatients with Hypertension under Treatment in Rural Communities

Peter Modupi Mphekgwana, Tebogo Maria Mothiba and Nancy Kgatla

Abstract

Hypertension is already a problem faced by South African urban populations, but little is known about the predominance, chance factors, and self-management strategies of hypertension in rural areas. Hypertension has an increased mortality and morbidity rate, thus has been identified as the killer disease in rural communities as its prevalence is increasing year by year. Non-attendance of hypertensive patients in rural communities has been identified as one of the most pressing issues in chronic illness, including hypertension, management and results into uncontrolled illnesses. Hypertensive patients lack self-management strategies to maintain their quality of life when diagnosed. Therefore, this book chapter is aimed at exploring the knowledge of self-management and strategies used in outpatients with hypertension under treatment in rural communities. Seven major themes were identified: paradoxical description; adherence to treatment and medication instructions, medical follow-up visits at the health facility, healthy lifestyle; management of emotions; defense mechanisms and religious interventions. Patients faced obstacles such as not eating a healthy diet since they are not the ones cooking, and children are always generating problems for them, leading their blood pressure and blood glucose levels to rise. Additional efforts are needed in rural communities to promote hypertension and self-management measures through educational programs.

Keywords: self-management, hypertension, non-communicable diseases (NCDs), cardiovascular disease (CVD), rural communities

1. Introduction

For centuries, communicable diseases have been responsible for the greatest worldwide burden of premature death. Following the Second World War, medical research achievements in the development of efficient and inexpensive vaccinations and the increased availability of antibiotics decreased the toll of communicable diseases even more [1]. Non-communicable diseases (NCDs) such as cardiovascular disease (CVD), diabetes, chronic-obstructive pulmonary disease (COPD), and cancers have emerged as an emerging pandemic with a major threat to the government. These diseases undermine health gains while imposing a heavy economic burden on governments and households worldwide in recent years [2, 3]. For example, according to the World Health Organization (WHO), NCDs are the leading cause of mortality worldwide, accounting for 71% of all deaths, with CVD accounting for the majority of deaths, with around 17.9 million people dying each year, followed by cancer, respiratory illnesses, and diabetes [4]. NCDs are the second leading cause of mortality in much of Sub-Saharan Africa (SSA), accounting for 2.6 million deaths [5]. Because of the rapidly expanding epidemic of NCDs, SSA is facing a double burden of NCD and communicable illnesses in a disadvantaged environment characterized by ill-health systems [6].

It is noted that CVD mortality rates are low in SSA as compared to high-income countries; however, the deaths due to CVD has doubled in the past three decades in SSA [7]. Certain risk factors, including hypertension and diabetes, are the key modifiable risk factors for poor CVD outcomes, such as stroke, the leading cause of death globally [7]. According to a study by Kearney et al. [8] using published literature from January 1, 1980, to December 31, 2002, the prevalence of hypertension was predicted to increase by about 60% to a total of 1·56 billion in the year 2025 [8]. The risk of hypertension in the semi-urban and rural areas of South Africa increases with age. It recorded 36% and 40% among the 56+ year population in semi-urban and rural areas, respectively [9]. Globally, including SSA, certain risk factors such as physical inactivity, family history of hypertension, unhealthy diets, waist-to-hip ratio (WHR), the harmful use of alcohol, and being diabetic are associated with hypertension [9–11]. Additionally, studies in Africa have shown that socio-economic status (SES), such as household wealth status and high BMI (overweight/obesity) is associated with hypertension [12, 13].

NCDs management includes diagnosing, screening for, and treating these illnesses and providing those in need with access to palliative care [4]. Undiagnosed hypertension in a rural district remains a concern. A large proportion of the hypertensive population remains undiagnosed, untreated, or inadequately treated in developing countries with most coming from lower socio-economic status (SES) than people with higher SES [12, 14]. If left undiagnosed and untreated in rural communities, this might increase the risk of a cardiovascular event, such as heart attack, stroke, enlarged heart, or kidney damage that may occur due to high blood pressure [11].

Most recent studies showed that community members had good (14%) or intermediate (74.3%) knowledge of hypertension, and only 11.8% of the population had poor knowledge even its risk factors [11, 15]. Lifestyle characteristics have direct correlations to hypertension risk, and modifying lifestyles in a favorable direction can significantly reduce hypertension risk [16]. However, poverty was highlighted as a key risk in this group, restricting healthy lifestyle choices and timely access to health treatment [15].

NCD management interventions are essential for achieving the global target of a 25% relative reduction in the risk of premature mortality from NCDs by 2025, and the sustainable development goal target of a one-third reduction in premature deaths from NCDs by 2030 [4]. Disease self-management, or patients' capacity to use disease information and engage in strategies that assist them in maintaining their health, helps lower death and hospitalization rates [17, 18]. Therefore, this chapter is aimed at exploring the knowledge of self-management and strategies in outpatients with hypertension under treatment in rural communities. We discuss risk factors for hypertension and discuss self-management strategies used by patients in rural communities.

2. Methodology

The study adopted a Mixed-Methods Research (MMR) approach, known as explanatory sequential design, advocated by Edmonds and Kennedy [19]. The study used a household administered data collecting tool in which quantitative data (QUAN) were collected through the non-laboratory INTERHEART risk score tool and qualitative data (QUAL) were obtained through semi-structured interviews. The data collection tool was distributed. The population eligible for this study was people staying in those selected rural communities and 18 years and above. Only 1224 completed the data collection tool with the assistance of community health workers (CHWs) using the non-laboratory INTERHEART risk score tool. For qualitative, participants were selected and interviewed until data saturation was reached. These respondents provided the qualitative data set that sought to explore the knowledge of self-management and strategies in outpatients with hypertension under treatment in rural communities. For quantitative data, frequencies were generated using the Statistical Programme for Social Sciences (SPPS version 26.0), and eight Steps of Tesch's inductive, descriptive open coding technique were used for qualitative data [20].

3. Quantitative phase

This section presents the demographic information of participants followed by risk levels findings. A standardized INTERHEART questionnaire instrument was employed in the study and 1244 individuals from a rural community in South Africa's Limpopo region responded (**Table 1**).

Of the 1244 participants, the majority were females (75%). In the majority of, participants their waist to hip ratio was less than 0.873 (54%). The median age of the participant was 48 years old. Regarding CVD risk factors status, 66% of adults in the rural area have hypertension while only 14% were diabetic, shown in **Figure 1**. Hypertension is more prevalent in rural communities than diabetes [21, 22]. However, there is substantial overlap between diabetes and hypertension, reflecting substantial overlap in their etiology and disease mechanisms [21]. Hypertension and diabetes are two of the leading risk factors for atherosclerosis and its complications, including heart attacks and strokes [23]. Making certain lifestyle changes (quit the smoke, drinking alcohol only in moderation, limiting salt intake, and eating a diet with low sugar but plenty of fruits, vegetables, fish, healthy fats, and whole grains) cannot only reduce complications from diabetes but can also greatly reduce your risk of high blood pressure [23]. The majority of the participants were non-smokers (89%) with 25% and 8% being hypertensive and diabetes, respectively.

Table 2 summarizes the quantitative data on the characteristics of rural community members in South Africa for hypertensive and non-hypertensive patients. Most participants in the study were females. Factors such as being female, hypertensive, and having comorbidity were associated with high risk developing coronary heart disease in the elderly than in younger patients [24]. The majority of the 175 (25%) hypertensive individuals in the study were at moderate risk of developing coronary heart disease.

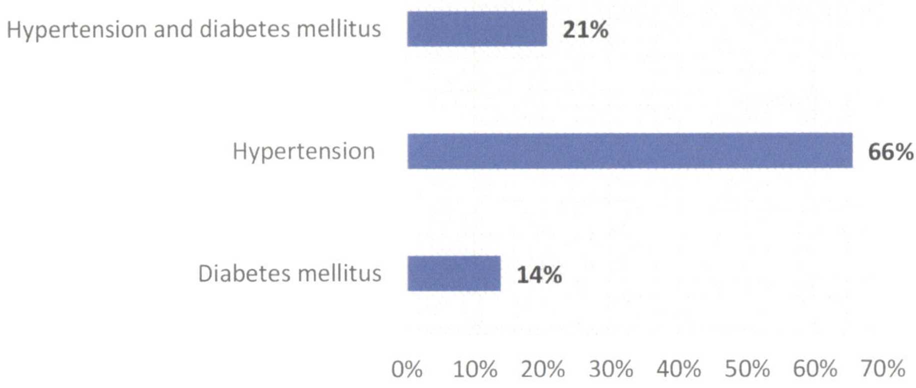

Figure 1.
Prime risk factor for cardiovascular disease.

Variables		**Median**	**95% CI (lower; upper)**
Age	Age	48	(47; 49)
Variables		Frequency	%
Gender	Male	306	25
	Female	918	75
Waist to hip ratio	Quartile 1: less than 0.873	654	54
	Quartile 2 & 3: 0.873–0.963	395	33
	Quartile 4: greater than or = 0.964	163	13
Smoking status	Current smoker	97	8
	Former smoker	38	3
	Non-smoker	1051	89
Hypertension	Yes	175	25
Diabetes	Yes	91	8

Table 1.
Characteristics of 1244 rural community members in South Africa.

4. Qualitative phase

Thematic analysis was applied to derive themes for discussion in this section. The following themes emerged: (1) paradoxical description of self-management strategies and (2) unforeseen painful life experiences.

4.1 Theme 1: paradoxical description of self-management strategies

The findings revealed that there is a different description of self-management strategies used by patients when living with risk factors such as hypertension. The strategies include engaging in physical activity, eating a healthy balanced diet, drinking a lot of water. However, the findings further indicate that most participants perform mild exercises and a limited number perform moderate exercises. Health promotion, self-care, and

Variables		Hypertensive 175 (25%)	Non-hypertensive
Age	Age	48 (20;94)	48 (18; 94)
Variables			
Gender	Male	41 (24%)	126 (25%)
	Female	131 (76%)	387 (75%)
Waist to hip ratio	Quartile 1: less than 0.873	71 (41%)	301 (59%)
	Quartile 2 & 3: 0.873–0.963	68 (39%)	152 (30%)
	Quartile 4: greater than or =0.964	34 (20%)	57 (11%)
Smoking status	Current smoker	11 (7%)	41 (8%)
	Former smoker	4 (2%)	25 (5%)
	Non-smoker	154 (91%)	442 (87%)
Risk of developing CVD	High	67 (39%)	24 (5%)
	Moderate	85 (49%)	159 (31%)
	Low	21 (12%)	332 (64%)

Table 2.
Descriptive characteristics of rural community members in South Africa for hypertensive and non-hypertensive patients.

education in the community and primary care settings have been shown to encourage patients to engage in smoking cessation, increased physical activity, and a healthy diet in the prevention of cardiovascular diseases, and this plays an important role in preventing CVD risk factors [16]. The stakeholders (health-care providers, health facilities, agencies involved in diabetes care, etc.) should encourage patients to understand the importance of diet, which may help in disease management, appropriate self-care and better quality of life. It is crucial to enhance basic diabetic and hypertension management and knowledge among the general population, especially in rural areas. National-level education and health intervention programs should be instigated and augmented.

4.1.1 Knowledge related to self-management strategies

It was seen that the majority of the participants indicated that physical activity, diet, and lifestyle modification are not associated with hypertension prevention. Most patients lack sufficient knowledge about NCDs and have little knowledge about physical activity [25]. It was discovered that time constraints, lack of interest, low self-esteem, lack of awareness, safety, and financial constraints, knowledge deficit, parental influence, peer pressure, and poverty were the barriers to physical activity and NCDs risk factors [25]. Knowledge plays a vital role in future disease development and early prevention and detection. Positive knowledge, attitude, and practice are important for hypertensive patients, and weight reduction should be considered in managing blood pressure [26, 27]. Knowledge, attitudes, and practices are interrelated and dependent on each other [27]. If the level of one element is higher, the other two factors should be affected positively. Knowledge regarding diabetes and hypertension varies greatly depending on socio-economic conditions, cultural beliefs and habits [27].

4.1.2 Adherence to treatment and medication instructions

Patients with hypertension on treatment are encouraged to adhere to prescribed treatment and medication instructions as this will assist in controlling the symptoms and promote quality of life. Adherence to treatment is described by Burnier and Egan as an important aspect that controls the symptoms which might be unbearable lead to complications [28]. Health professionals who include physicians, pharmacists and nurses assist in making sure that patients improve and adhere to treatment. Additionally, though adherence to treatment and medical instructions is important, hypertensive patients are further advised to manage their lifestyle because that reduces the risk of developing CVDs and improves clinical outcomes.

4.1.3 Adherence to medical follow up visits at the health facility

It is important to emphasise adherence to medical follow-up scheduled dates because during such a visit, the health professionals teach patients about various issues, including all self-care strategies and pharmacological interventions that are equally effective.

4.1.4 Adherence to a healthy lifestyle and lifestyle modification

The hypertensive patients are encouraged to make sure that they adhere to a healthy lifestyle which includes lifestyle modifications that require more effort to do that. A healthy lifestyle includes a healthy diet, exercise, have resting times, etc. [29].

4.1.5 Management of emotions (anger, fear, stress) is outlined as a self-management strategy

The importance of managing emotions such as depression, anxiety, excessive worry, anger, fear, and stress needs to be emphasised when interacting with hypertensive patients. When they experience such, they must consult health professionals for help [30].

4.1.6 Defence mechanisms

Hypertensive patients are encouraged to use the self-defence mechanism because this assists one to cope with all life's negative situations leading to minimal symptoms of the disease [31].

4.1.7 Religious interventions

Religious beliefs and practices are viewed as a method to assist people in adjusting to their situations and the physical, mental, and social difficulties brought about by clinical disease [32].

4.2 Theme 2: unforeseen painful life experiences

According to the findings, there is an explanation for how unforeseen painful life experiences lead to inadequate management or avoidance of risk variables. For example, hypertension and diabetes-mellitus, as most of the participants indicated that they experience challenges like not adhering to a healthy diet as they are not the ones cooking. Children are always causing problems to them that cause their blood pressure and blood glucose to increase. As a result of a lack of support for family care from health services and professionals, family vulnerability is formed or exacerbated because family potential decreases over time due to care needs, which are continually refreshed and augmented in chronic diseases [33]. In both the genesis and the potential of overcoming vulnerabilities, it appears that family support in the experience of disease and caregiving might be a crucial factor [33]. Medical illiteracy among patients (i.e., poor understanding of the disease process, medication effects, dosage regimens, and possible side effects) is a frequent cause of medication non-adherence, leading to painful experiences. The majority of uncontrolled hypertension is due to poor adherence to antihypertensive medications [34]. Understanding the types of causes that contribute to noncompliance helps address noncompliance.

5. Integration phase

Quantitative investigation	**Qualitative investigation**	
Quantitative findings	**Sub-themes**	**Participants expression**
67.8% and 79.9% of survey respondents with hypertension reported consuming enough fruits and vegetables daily, respectively. 66% and 61.5% of survey respondents with hypertension reported eating meat and salty food one or more times a day. 25.9% of survey respondents with hypertension perform moderate physical activity in my leisure time	Paradoxical description of self-management strategies (physical activity, eating a healthy balanced diet, drinking a lot of water, etc.) *1.1. Knowledge related to self-management strategies*	This is supported by the following The other participants added how she manages herself HP#02:- *To prevent CVD I don't take too much sugar, and also I use a small amount of salt, and for meat, I eat chicken only I don't eat beef as is the one that causes a problem. When I was still working, I used to buy vegetables and fruits but now is bad because to buy with pension money I can't afford those things, but I use traditional vegetables is very healthy. The vegetables that I use are potatoes and fish because I can afford them.*
38.5% of survey respondents with hypertension showed to be at a high risk of coronary heart disease	*1.2 Adherence to treatment & medication instructions*	The findings were also supported by participant HP#04:- *I manage myself by just taking treatment as instructed although I don't know whether I'm preventing heart attack, I think by taking treatment and adhering to a diet of avoiding salts and fats I think my body and heart will flow normally and prevent heart attacks.*
	1.3 Adherence to medical follow up visits at the health facility	Participant HP#08:- *I think they should follow clinic instructions by taking treatment as prescribed and take too much water to dilute high blood and also to take fruits and vegetables as they protect your body and also to avoid sleeping a lot as high blood needs an active person do house chores as high blood is not life-threatening illness is everybody's sickness we are not supposed to fear it.*
	1.4 Adherence to a healthy lifestyle & lifestyle modification	Participant HP# 04:- *I manage myself by making sure I eat a healthy meal, you see my wife died in 2015 and I'm left with 4 children all of them are taking care of me, you see I'm wearing Adidas clothes and shoes I'm well taken care of. In the case of diet, I'm taking too many vegetables and fruits because as I stay alone, but I have many chickens well protected in a fence I eat those chickens because they are healthy, unlike the ones from the fridge because they cause painful leg.*

Quantitative investigation	Qualitative investigation	
Quantitative findings	**Sub-themes**	**Participants expression**
33.3% of survey respondents with hypertension felt work or home life stress in the last year	*1.5 Management of emotions (anger, fear, stress) mentioned as a self-management strategy*	Participants HP# 010 highlighted that: - *Many things that can contribute to CVD is by thinking too much and also became angry on small issues you know sometimes as a human being people can make you angry or hurt you very deep that it can take time to heal and forget and you unable to let it go this can also cause CVD.*
2.3% of survey respondents with hypertension were former smokers	*1.6 Defence mechanisms*	Participant HP# 03 confirmed by saying: - *Myself is long I have been taking treatment since 2008 but, due to exercising I'm always healthy and energetic, my day starts with cleaning the whole yard which is a very huge yard thereafter I clean the house, wash dishes and cook my meal you can undermine this but is a very serious exercise.*
	1.7 Religious interventions	This is supported by participant HP#015:- *I make sure I eat healthy foods and avoid smoking and alcohol like when I fast I make sure that I eat once in a day not fasting all day as I may faint and feel dizzy and praying God helps to connect you with the holy spirit that will lead you and be relieved in your body and spirit.*

Table 3.
Integration of the quantitative and qualitative results.

Integration of the QUAN and QUAL results revealed that most of the patients are engaging in eating a healthy balanced diet (**Table 3**). QUAN results pointed out that more than 61% of outpatients were consuming enough fruits and vegetables daily but still eating meat and salty food one or more times a day and physical inactivity. Combining the eating plan and a lower salt consumption could provide the most effective and may reduce hypertension risk [35]. It is observed that patients still consume high salts and a lot of meat on daily basis, however, some reported that they avoid eating beef meat as compared to chicken meat and also, try to use a small amount of salt and sugar. Patients adhere to treatment and medication instructions and medical follow-up visits at the health facility as other self-management ways of hypertension. The proper use of antihypertensive medications is a critical component of hypertension management [36]. Knowledge of hypertension and its treatment, socio-demographics, treatment views, and patient-provider interaction may contribute to poor drug adherence [36]. Poor adherence might worsen diseases and increase the likelihood of cardiovascular events such as heart attack or a stroke. Most hypertensive patients in rural areas are adherent to medication and clinic visits, however, about 39% of patients were at a high risk of coronary heart disease.

It is observed that about 33% felt work or home life stress. A stressful situation leads to a surge of hormones and temporarily increases your blood pressure. Although stress does not directly cause hypertension, it does trigger a rush of hormones and momentarily raises your blood pressure, which may later develop into hypertension [37]. Some hypertensive patients reported managing their emotions by avoiding stress, overthinking, and becoming angry as a self-management strategy. Most patients, especially pensioners and the elderly, perform household duties every morning and clean the yard, which they believe is adequate because they have large yards. Risk behaviors such as smoking and alcohol use have direct correlations to hypertension risk, and avoiding such risk behaviors can significantly reduce hypertension risk [9–11]. Due to religious interventions, some patients eat healthy foods and avoid smoking and alcohol.

6. Conclusion

Hypertensive patients residing in rural communities seem to lack sufficient knowledge concerning hypertension self-management strategies. Additional efforts are needed in rural communities to promote hypertension and self-management measures through educational programs such as encouraging patients to engage in increased physical activity and a healthy diet.

Acknowledgements

The authors would like to thank all participants, notably community health workers, professional nurses in clinics, SPICES research participants, the University of Limpopo, and the Limpopo Provincial Department of Health. Finally, we would like to express our gratitude to the European Commission for sponsoring this initiative.

Author details

Peter Modupi Mphekgwana[1*], Tebogo Maria Mothiba[2] and Nancy Kgatla[3]

1 Department of Research Administration and Development, University of Limpopo, Polokwane, South Africa

2 Faculty of Health Science, University of Limpopo, Polokwane, South Africa

3 Department of Nursing Science, University of Limpopo, Polokwane, South Africa

*Address all correspondence to: peter.mphekgwana@ul.ac.za

References

[1] Holmes KK, Bertozzi S, Bloom BR, Jha P, Gelband H, DeMaria LM, et al. Major infectious diseases: Key messages from disease control priorities. Major Infectious Diseases. 2017

[2] Terzic A, Waldman S. Chronic diseases: The emerging pandemic. Clinical and Translational Science. 2011;**4**(3):225-226

[3] Burki TK. WHO releases latest report on the global tobacco epidemic. The Lancet Oncology. 2021 Sep 1;**22**(9):1217

[4] World Health Organization. WHO package of essential noncommunicable (PEN) disease interventions for primary health care

[5] Yuyun MF, Sliwa K, Kengne AP, Mocumbi AO, Bukhman G. Cardiovascular diseases in Sub-Saharan Africa compared to high-income countries: An epidemiological perspective. Global Heart. 2020;**15**(1)

[6] Boutayeb A, Boutayeb S. The burden of non communicable diseases in developing countries. International Journal for Equity in Health. 2005;**4**(1):1-8

[7] Afshin A, Sur PJ, Fay KA, Cornaby L, Ferrara G, Salama JS, et al. Health effects of dietary risks in 195 countries, 1990-2017: A systematic analysis for the Global Burden of Disease Study 2017. The Lancet. 2019;**393**(10184):1958-1972

[8] Kearney PM, Whelton M, Reynolds K, Muntner P, Whelton PK, He J. Global burden of hypertension: Analysis of worldwide data. The Lancet. 2005;**365**(9455):217-223

[9] Mphekgwana PM, Malema N, Monyeki KD, Mothiba TM, Makgahlela M, Kgatla N, et al. Hypertension prevalence and determinants among Black South African adults in semi-urban and rural areas. International Journal of Environmental Research and Public Health. 2020;**17**(20):7463

[10] Bokaba M, Modjadji P, Mokwena KE. Undiagnosed hypertension in a workplace: The case of a logistics company in Gauteng, South Africa. Healthcare. 2021;**9**(8):964

[11] Princewel F, Cumber SN, Kimbi JA, Nkfusai CN, Keka EI, Viyoff VZ, et al. Prevalence and risk factors associated with hypertension among adults in a rural setting: The case of Ombe, Cameroon. The Pan African Medical Journal [Internet]. 2019 Nov 14;**34**(147). Available from: https://www.ncbi.nlm.nih.gov/pmc/articles/PMC7025826/

[12] Sharma JR, Mabhida SE, Myers B, Apalata T, Nicol E, Benjeddou M, et al. Prevalence of hypertension and its associated risk factors in a rural Black population of Mthatha Town, South Africa. International Journal of Environmental Research and Public Health. 2021;**18**(3):1215

[13] Yaya S, El-Khatib Z, Ahinkorah BO, Budu E, Bishwajit G. Prevalence and socioeconomic factors of diabetes and high blood pressure among women in Kenya: A cross-sectional study. Journal of Epidemiology and Global Health. 2021;**16**:1-8

[14] Islam FM, Bhuiyan A, Chakrabarti R, Rahman MA, Kanagasingam Y, Hiller JE. Undiagnosed hypertension in a rural district in Bangladesh: The Bangladesh population-based Diabetes and Eye Study (BPDES). Journal of Human Hypertension. 2016;**30**(4):252-259

[15] Jongen VW, Lalla-Edward ST, Vos AG, Godijk NG, Tempelman H, Grobbee DE, et al. Hypertension in a rural community in South Africa: What they know, what they think they know and what they recommend. BMC Public Health. 2019;**19**(1) 1-0

[16] Budreviciute A, Damiati S, Sabir DK, Onder K, Schuller-Goetzburg P, Plakys G, et al. Management and prevention strategies for non-communicable diseases (NCDs) and their risk factors. Frontiers in Public Health. 2020;**26**(8):788

[17] Allegrante JP, Wells MT, Peterson JC. Interventions to support behavioral self-management of chronic diseases. Annual Review of Public Health. 2019;**1**(40):127-146

[18] Mothiba TM. Self-management strategies to curb the development of NCDs in rural communities. In: Lifestyle and Epidemiology: The Double Burden of Poverty and Cardiovascular Diseases in African Populations. IntechOpen; 2021 Mar 19:285

[19] Edmonds WA, Kennedy TD. An Applied Guide to Research Designs: Quantitative, Qualitative, and Mixed Methods. Sage Publications; 20 April 2016

[20] Creswell JW, Creswell JD. Research Design: Qualitative, Quantitative, and Mixed Methods Approaches. Sage Publications; 27 Nov 2017

[21] Senanayake S, Ruwanpathirana T, Gunawardena N. Hypertension in a rural community in Sri Lanka: Prevalence, associated factors and its effect on the renal profile. Journal of Hypertension. 2019;**37**(9):1805-1812

[22] Malema RN, Mphekgwana PM, Makgahlela M, Mothiba TM, Monyeki KD, Kgatla N, et al. Community-based screening for cardiovascular disease in the Capricorn District of Limpopo Province, South Africa. The Open Public Health Journal. 10 Jun 2021;**14**(1):241-249

[23] Torp-Pedersen C, Jeppesen J. Diabetes and hypertension and atherosclerotic cardiovascular disease: Related or separate entities often found together. Hypertension. 2011;**57**(5):887-888

[24] Yayan J. Association of traditional risk factors with coronary artery disease in nonagenarians: The primary role of hypertension. Clinical Interventions in Aging. 2014;**9**:2003

[25] Onagbiye SO, Tshwaro RM, Barry A, Marie Y. Physical activity and non-communicable disease risk factors: Knowledge and perceptions of youth in a low resourced Community in the Western Cape. The Open Public Health Journal [Internet]. 2019 Dec 31;**12**(1):558-566. [cited Jun 16, 2021]

[26] Tahir Q, Azam N, Imran M, Hashmi A, Zeb A, Furqan A. Knowledge, attitudes and practices of patients regarding diabetes and hypertension control. Journal of Postgraduate Medical Institute (Peshawar-Pakistan). 2018;**32**(2):166-172

[27] Fatema K, Hossain S, Natasha K, Chowdhury HA, Akter J, Khan T, et al. Knowledge attitude and practice regarding diabetes mellitus among nondiabetic and diabetic study participants in Bangladesh. BMC Public Health. 2017;**17**(1) 1-0

[28] Burnier M, Egan BM. Adherence in hypertension: A review of prevalence, risk factors, impact, and management. Circulation Research. 2019;**124**(7):1124-1140

[29] Chuk P, Tsai A, Siu A, Tang V. Evaluating a healthy lifestyle training program for a group of China medical students. Clinical Health Promotion - Research and Best Practice for patients, staff and community. 2020;**10**(1):15-21

[30] Li W, Tian M. Exploring emotion management strategies of junior high school teachers in Shanghai, China. In: Emotion Management and Feelings in Teaching and Educational Leadership. Emerald Publishing Limited; 28 May 2019

[31] Van Smoorenburg AN, Hertroijs DF, Dekkers T, Elissen AM, Melles M. Patients' perspective on self-management: Type 2 diabetes in daily life. BMC Health Services Research. 2019;**19**(1):1-8

[32] He FX, Turnbull B, Kirshbaum MN, Phillips B, Klainin-Yobas P. Assessing stress, protective factors and psychological well-being among undergraduate nursing students. Nurse Education Today. 2018;**1**(68):4-12

[33] Bellato R, Araújo LF, Dolina JV, Musquim CD, Corrêa GH. The family experience of care in chronic situation. Revista da Escola de Enfermagem da USP. 2016;**50**:81-88

[34] Vrijens B, Antoniou S, Burnier M, de la Sierra A, Volpe M. Current situation of medication adherence in hypertension. Frontiers in Pharmacology. 2017; **1**(8):100

[35] Juraschek SP, Miller ER, Weaver CM, Appel LJ. Effects of sodium reduction and the DASH diet in relation to baseline blood pressure. Journal of the American College of Cardiology. 2017;**70**(23):2841-2848

[36] Van der Feltz-Cornelis CM, Van Oppen P, Van Marwijk HW, De Beurs E, Van Dyck R. A patient–doctor relationship questionnaire (PDRQ-9) in primary care: Development and psychometric evaluation. General Hospital Psychiatry. 2004;**26**(2):115-120

[37] Kulkarni S, O'Farrell I, Erasi M, Kochar MS. Stress and hypertension. WMJ: official publication of the State Medical Society of Wisconsin. 1998;**97**(11):34-38

Chapter 6

Sodium and Potassium Nutritional Status Provides a New View on the Essential Hypertension

Berislav Momčilović

Abstract

Short-term biological indicator of urinary Na and K excretion is generally used to assess Na and K dietary exposure. In this study, we used the long-term biological indicator of hair to assess Na and K nutritional status. Hair Na and K were analyzed in 1073 healthy adult white Caucasians [734 women (♀) and 339 men (♂)] with the ICP MS. The log-transformed data were analyzed with median derivatives bioassay. The median values (μg•g^{-1}) were ♀Na 254 and ♂Na 371, and ♀K 74.3 and ♂K 143, respectively. The linear (adequate) ranges of the sigmoid saturation curve ranges for sodium were ♀Na 55.6–1307 and ♂Na 84.0–1450, whereas these ranges for potassium were ♀K 18.9–467 and ♂K 25.8–1079. The strict homeostatic control of whole blood K and Na renders them unsuitable for assessing the nutritional status. The potassium to sodium ratio (K/Na) in women appears stable across the sigmoid linear segment range, contrary to the constantly increasing K/Na ratio in Men. The results suggest that hair Na concentration should not be below 55.6 and 84.0 or above 1307 and 1450 μg•g-1 in women and men, respectively. Similarly, K hair concentrations should not be below 18.0 and 25.8 and higher than 46.7 and 107.9 in women and men, respectively. Hair K/Na ratio should stay about 0.600 in M and 0.400 in W. Current dietary salt exposure of the general US population does not require preventive across the board salt restriction.

Keywords: potassium, sodium, hair, whole blood, nutritional status, essential hypertension

1. Introduction

Sodium and potassium are the principal extracellular and intracellular cationic elements of the human body, respectively [1]. However, the link between habitual salt dietary intake and general public health is still controversial [2]. Over the last decades, a plethora of studies informed us how excess dietary salt is associated with hypertension and cerebral stroke [3–5]. That leads to the recent draconian recommendations for the general population for the dietary salt restriction [6]. However, the deeply echeloned crusade against what is now the habitual dietary salt intake is strongly criticized because of the flaws of many studies statistical design and "cherry picking" of the data [7], that the basic tenants of the human physiology were either ignored or misinterpreted [8] and that there were too much bureaucratic political meddling in the salt restriction issues [9].

The simple idea on how the reduction of sodium dietary intake may be a health protection measure for the general population to prevent the development of hypertension and cerebral stroke is certainly a very appealing one. That idea has been tested by a waste number of authors who studied the relationship between blood pressure and dietary sodium and potassium intake and their urinary excretion (separately or in combination), and what comprehensive review is beyond the aim of this article. Indeed, there are difficulties associated with the timing and assessing of the correct blood pressure readings [10], the problem with the control of the complex variability of the tested dietary composition [11, 12], and the problems on how to adequately assess the dietary intake of either sodium and potassium [13, 14].

The aim of this research is to assess sodium and potassium nutritional status by analyzing their frequency distribution in the hair and whole blood of adult men and women with a median derivatives bioassay [15]. Today, a century-old dictum "We are what we eat" may be modified to run "Hair knows what we eat" [16]. Indeed, hair is the long-term biological indicator of the bioelement nutritional status, whereas the current "golden standard" of the urine is a short-term biological indicator [17]. It should be noted that we used the term "bioelement" as a common denominator for the major elements (electrolytes) like Na and K, trace elements like I and Se, and ultra-trace elements like Cr and Ni [15].

2. Subjects and methods

This prospective, observational, cross-sectional, and the exploratory epidemiological study was approved by the Ethical Committee of the Institute for Research and Development of the Sustainable Eco Systems (IRES), Zagreb, Croatia. The study was conducted in adherence to the Declaration of Helsinki on Human Subject Research [18]. Every subject gave his/her written consent to participate in the study and filled out a short questionnaire on his/her health status and medical history (data not shown) [19]. Data on hair shampooing were also recorded and none of them declared the presence of elements under the observation.

Hair potassium and sodium were analyzed in a random sample of 1073 apparently healthy white Caucasian adults (339 men, 734 women). Whole blood K and Na were analyzed in a subset of 212 subjects (143 women and 91 men); the median age of women and men was 47 and 50 years, respectively. Our population consisted of subjects from the general Croatian population who were interested to learn more about their health status; the majority of them were living in the capital city region of Zagreb, Croatia. All the subjects consumed their usual home-prepared mixed mid-European diet, and none of them have reported an adverse medical health condition.

Hair K and Na and whole blood K and Na were analyzed with the inductively coupled plasma mass spectrometry (ICP-MS, Elan 9000, Perkin Elmer, Canada) at the Center for Biotic Medicine (CBM), Moscow, Russia. The CBM is an ISO Europe certified commercial laboratory for analyzing bioelements (electrolytes, trace elements, and ultra-trace elements) in different biological matrices in health and disease. CBM is also a member of the exclusive External Quality Assessment of the UK Surrey scientific group for the quality control of trace element analysis. Hair K and Na analyses were performed following the International Atomic Energy Agency recommendations [20] and other validated analytical methods and procedures [21].

Preparation of hair and whole blood for the ICP-MS analysis is described in Appendix A, Part A for the hair and Part B for the whole blood. The detection limits for K and Na in the hair were 4.3 ppm for Na and 0.3 ppm for K, and in the whole blood, they were 0.6 ppm for Na and 0.04 for K. All chemicals were of pro analysis grade (Khimmed Sintez, Moscow, Russia).

To scrutinize the respective hair and whole blood potassium and sodium concentration frequency distribution, we used the median derivative bioassay of the log-transformed data, to fit the sigmoid logistic regression function (power function) [22] for men and women separately (Appendices B and C)

$$A2 + (A1–A2)/[1 + (x/x0)p] \quad (1)$$

Where A1 is the initial value (lower horizontal asymptote), A2 is the final value (upper horizontal asymptote), x0 is the center (point of inflection) is the median (M_0 detected), p is power (the parameter that affects the slope of the area about the inflection point). The OriginPro 8.0 data analysis and graphing software was used for this analysis (OriginLab Corp., OriginPro Version 8.0., Northampton, MA).

The hair deposition of a K and Na below the linear segment range of the sigmoid saturation curve denotes a deficient hair uptake of K and Na; when their concentration is within the linear range segment that indicates a safe and adequate hair K and Na uptake, and when K and Na concentrations are above the linear range segment of the sigmoid power curve, that denotes the excessive level of their hair uptake [23]. The central adequate linear segment of the sigmoid power curve may be further subdivided into low adequate, safe, and supra-adequate segments with a 60:30:10 ratio [17], but some other ratios, like 30:60:10 ratio, may be also considered. It is well known that our body may adapt to a given nutrient intake so that balanced nutrition can occur at various dietary levels of the nutrients. Thus, sparse diets are not necessarily deficient ones, although they often are [23].

3. Results

To correct for the exponential pattern of the data distribution, we log-transformed the potassium and sodium hair and whole body concentration data for men and women separately. Such a data transformation generated a classical Gaussian bell-shaped frequency distribution. Hair potassium data frequency distribution for both men and women is shown in the upper left part of **Figure 1,** whereas the data for sodium frequency distribution is shown in the lower left part of the same figure. The hair of both men and women has higher concentrations of sodium than potassium. Indeed, hair sodium median concentrations were ($\mu g\ g^{-1}$) 371.5 for men (M, ♂) and 254 for women (W, ♀), whereas the comparative hair potassium concentrations were lower for both M•K 142.5 and W•K 73.7 (**Figure 2A**). The median potassium to sodium ratio (K/Na R) was 0.385 for M and 0.298 for W, respectively (**Table 1**).

Similarly, whole blood (WB) concentrations were also higher for sodium than potassium (**Figure 3A**). WB medians for sodium were M•Na 178 and W•Na 181 $\mu g\ g^{-1}$, whereas WB potassium medians were M•K 1369 and W•K 1324, respectively. The K/Na median ratios were M•K/Na 0.769 and W•K/Na 0,731and they were almost identical with the overlapping CV intervals. It should be noted that WB potassium

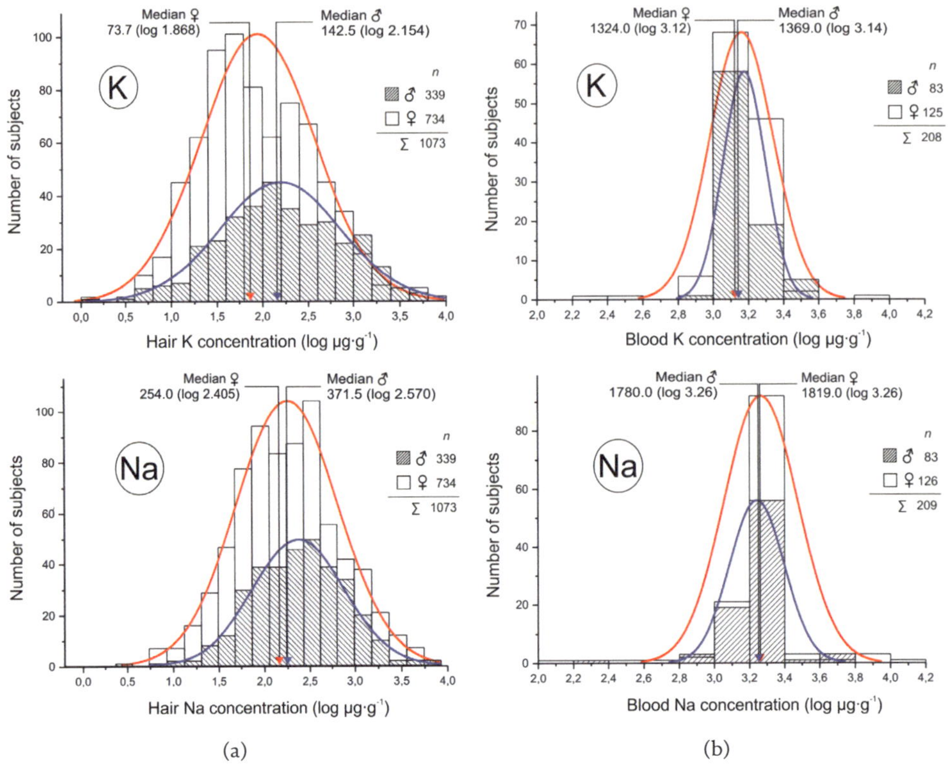

Figure 1.
(a) Left hair K and Na cumulative distribution in women ( ) and men ( ) (log µg g⁻¹). (b) Right whole blood K and Na cumulative distribution in women ( ) and men ( ) (log µg g⁻¹).

Gaussian distribution showed a tendency of slightly leaning to the right, whereas, contrary to that, sodium showed a tendency to lean to the left, which indicates subtle sex potassium and sodium metabolic differences.

Our median derivatives bioassay allowed for the transformation of the Gaussian bell-shaped frequency distribution curves for hair potassium and sodium into their sigmoid saturation curves (**Figure 2A** for K and **Figure 2B** for Na). The numerical data for the shown median derivatives points are presented within Appendix C.1 for potassium and Appendix C.2 for Sodium. The sigmoid saturation curves started being linear at the median derivative points W•d3 and M•D3 but the linear upward trend started earlier in women than in men. However, the linear segments for both men and women sigmoid saturation curves for hair potassium would fuse together again at the median derivatives upward point of W•u3 and M•U3. However, the linear medium derivatives range segments for hair sodium get merged much earlier for W at u1 and for M at U1, respectively. We assume that the observed suggests a tighter metabolic control of sodium than potassium in both men and women.

The median derivatives bioassay data for whole blood (WB) generated almost vertical steep and narrow linear ranges for both men (**Figure 3A**) and women (**Figure 3B**). Indeed, the linear segments of the median derivatives between men and women for the same bioelement were almost identical. However, potassium and sodium WB concentrations were both higher in men than women. The data demonstrated impressively tight homeostatic control of WB sodium and potassium for both

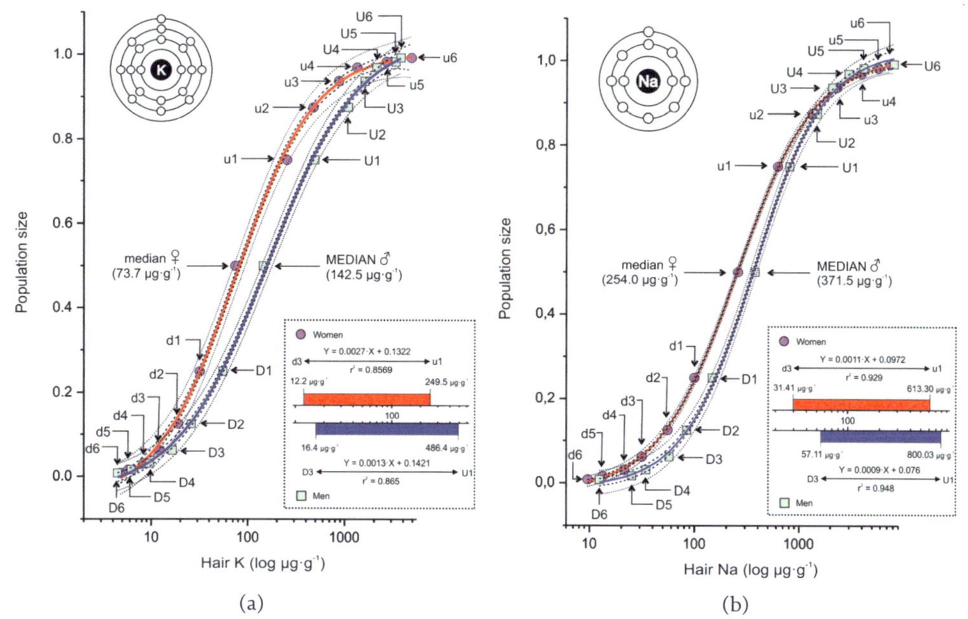

Figure 2.
(a) Hair potassium median derivatives bioassay. Men n = 339 ( ) and Women n = 73 ( ). D, U men downward (D) and upward (U) median derivatives; d, u women downward (d) and upward (u) median derivatives. — Logistic function $Y = A2 + (A1–A2)/(1 + (X/X_0)^P)$, - - - 0.95 confidence limit, ••• 0.95 prediction limit. Men: $Y = 1.045 + (–0.040 – 1.045)/(1 + (X/151.62)^{0.934})$, $r^2 = 0.999$; Women: $Y = 1.006 + (–0.059 – 1.006)/(1 + (X/74.03)^{1.065})$, $r^2 = 0.999$. BOX: Potassium linear saturation range for and (log conc). See Appendix A for the Median derivatives bioassay model and Appendix B for median derivatives bioassay model input values. (b) Hair sodium derivatives bioassay. Men n = 339 ( ) and women n = 734 ( ). D, U men downward (D) and upward (U) median derivatives; d, u Women downward (d) and upward (u) median derivatives. — Logistic function $Y = A2 + (A1–A2)/(1 + (X/X_0)^P)$, - - - 0.95 confidence limit, ••• 0.95 prediction limit. Men: $Y = 1.025 + (–0.011 – 1.025)/(1 + (X/363.95)^{1.302})$, $r^2 = 0.999$; Women: $Y = 1.008 + (-0.018 – 1.008)/(1 + (X/247.73)^{1.179})$, $r^2 = 0.999$. BOX: Sodium linear saturation range for and (log conc). See Appendix A for the Median derivatives bioassay model and Appendix B for median derivatives bioassay models input values.

	Men			Women		
	Minimum (D2)	Median (U2)	Maximum (U2)	Minimum (d2)	Median (u2)	Maximum (u2)
Potassium	10.3	155.9	1100.5	20.6	81.6	483.9
Sodium	91.2	364.3	1577.3	60.9	275.9	1377.2
K/Na	0.113	0.420	0.698	0.337	0.296	0.337

Table 1.
Potassium/Sodium ratio of the linear part of the sigmoid saturation curve ($\mu g\ g^{-1}$).

sexes. Such a tight control implies poor WB adequacy in assessing both Na and K dietary intake impact

We also directly cross-compared the relationship of hair Na and K concentrations over their median derivatives linear range (**Figure 4**). Apparently, there is a difference in K and Na quantitative saturation along with the hair fiber. Since even the sparse diets may be nutritionally adequate, it is reasonable to assume that the initial linear part of the sigmoid saturation curve presents the subclinical or low adequate

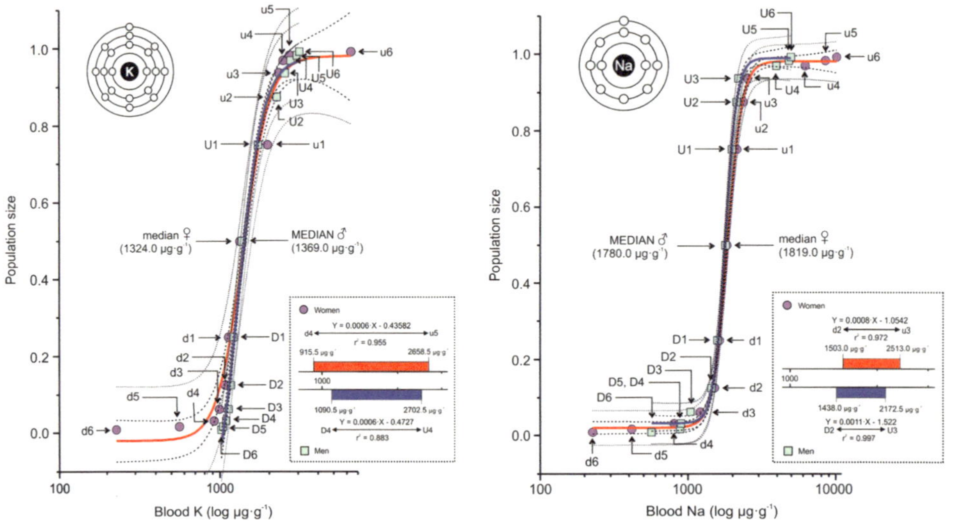

(a) (b)

Figure 3.
(a) Whole blood potassium median derivatives bioassay. Men n = 83 ( ) and women n = 125 ( ). D, U men downward (D) and upward (U) median derivatives; d, u Women downward (d) and upward (u) median derivatives. — Logistic function $Y = A2 + (A1-A2)/(1 + (X/X_0)^p)$, *- - - 0.95 confidence limit, ••• 0.95 prediction limit. Men:* $Y = 0.976 + (-0.289 - 0.976)/(1 + (X/1293.56)^{5.751})$, $r^2 = 0.992$; *Women:* $Y = 0.981 + (-0.021 - 0.981)/(1 + (X/1392.17)^{5.505})$, $r^2 = 0.981$. *BOX: Potassium linear saturation range for and (log conc). See Appendix A for the Median derivatives bioassay model and Appendix B for the Median derivatives bioassay input values. (b) Whole blood sodium median derivatives bioassay. Men n = 83 ( ) and Women n = 126 ( ). D, U Men downward (D) and upward (U) median derivatives; d, u Women downward (d) and upward (u) median derivatives. — Logistic function* $Y = A2 + (A1-A2)/(1 + (X/X_0)^p)$, *- - - 0.95 confidence limit, ••• 0.95 prediction limit. Men:* $Y = 0.989 + (0.032 - 0.989)/(1 + (X/1772.25)^{11.171})$, $r^2 = 0.997$; *women:* $Y = 0.981 + (0.019 - 0.981)/(1 + (X/1843.34)^{8.959})$, $r^2 = 0.998$. *BOX: Sodium linear saturation range for and (log conc). See Appendix A for the model and Appendix B for median derivatives input values.*

nutritional response range. Alternatively, the 30–90% segment of the sigmoid curve linear range represents a truly adequate K and Na dietary intake range. Interestingly enough, the correlation coefficient r^2 was impressively high for individual potassium and sodium slopes, i.e., r^2 for M•Na was 0.948 and that for W•Na was 0.929 whereas r^2 for M•K it was 0.865 and W•K was 0.857. However, when comparative data for hair sodium were plotted on the X-axis, and potassium data on Y-axis, the combined r^2 correlation coefficient dropped to 0.487. These data indicate that there is a considerable capacity for homeostatic adaptation within the hair follicle to the changes in the available circulating amounts of dietary Na and K. Apparently, the constant and efficient homeostatic control of Na and K in the whole blood is accompanied by their highly variable concentrations in the hair which acts as a river lavvy for water excess.

Collected data showed a tempting impression of how hair Na tends to increase with aging whereas hair K tends to decrease over the same time period (**Figure 4**). Indeed, there was a significant age-dependent increase of sodium in the hair of women ($p < 0.05$, Pearson's coefficient), but not in men. Presumably, the number of our men was too small to conclusively show the presumed age-dependent increase of hair Na in men. Or we may be dealing with a problem of the statistical inequality in the mathematical statistics. All in all, the data showed some reflex on sarcopenia, i.e., age-dependent muscle loss in old age, and failure in the control of sodium in old age.

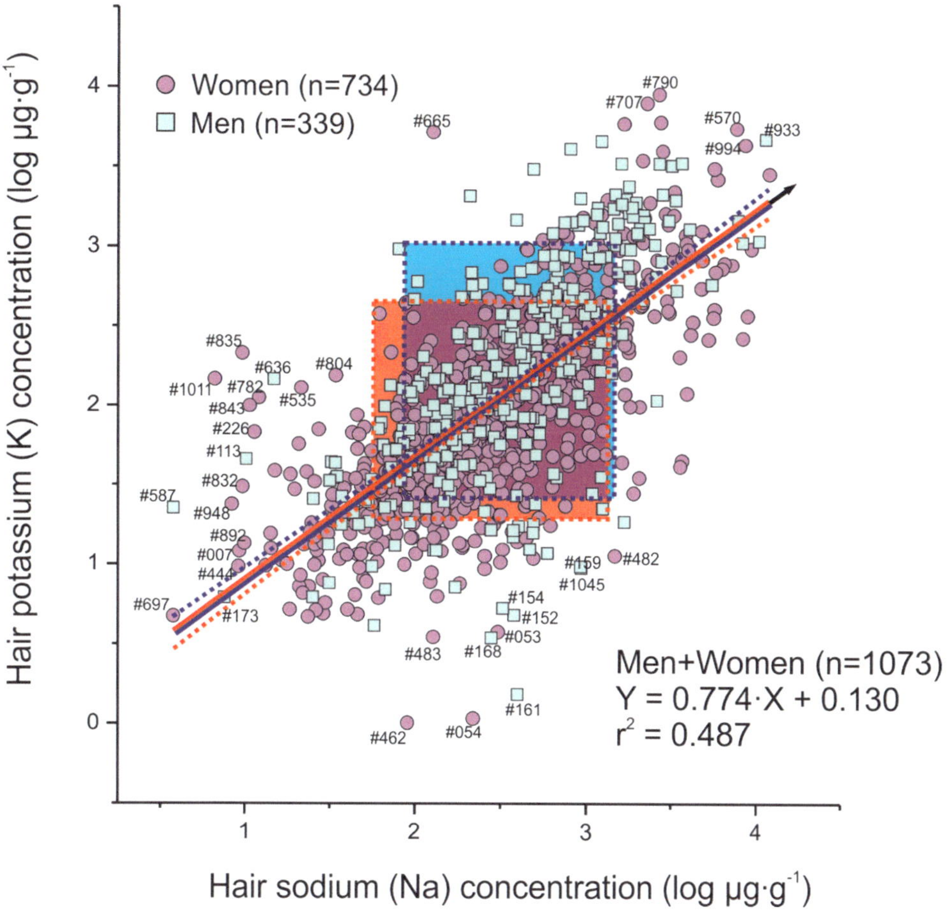

Figure 4.
Hair potassium/sodium (K/Na) ratio. The squared region over the regression line covers a 30–90% of the adequate nutritional status. Internal red square: women, internal blue square: men.

4. Discussion

Human hair makes a valuable long-term biological indicator tissue for the assessment of the nutritional status of the essential bioelements [17, 24, 25]. Hair growth is a unidirectional process that, in difference to urine, precludes sodium and potassium post absorption metabolic equilibration with the surrounding organs and tissues of the human body [15]. Indeed, the results of our study demonstrated that the human nutritional status of potassium and sodium may be adequately assessed with the hair median derivatives bioassay. This median derivatives bioassay generates from the body of the collected data set and not by subjecting the data to some external preconceived model upon them, i.e., not from the data themselves. Indeed, the median derivatives bioassay relies upon the central part of the Gaussian statistical data distribution curve, i.e., on its linear segment when the data were log-transformed. This is a substantial difference in comparison to the standard statistical approach where we are focused on the data distribution tails. Indeed, the linear segment of the sigmoid curve covers for entire one standard deviation of the entire population data set. Moreover, the median derivatives bioassay model avoids the problem of J-shaped curves transformation [26] and other problems associated with the no threshold assumption linear regression model [27].

This study revealed subtle gender-dependent metabolic differences in the homeostatic control of sodium and potassium metabolism. Both Na and K belong to the first column of the periodic system and they are entangled in the control of the cell membrane ionic Na and K transport. In our study, the bio entangled K/Na ratio stays constant over the linear (adequate) part of the sigmoid saturation curve in women but progressively increases in men. We already know that the increased intake of potassium suppresses the appearance of hypertension induced by the increased sodium dietary exposure [28]. Apparently, being a man carries the inherited risk towards development of the hypertension.

Today, an average adult American `men and women aged 19–71+ years are consuming 2.83–3.34 and 2.21–2.43 mg K per day, respectively. At the same time, the average daily consumption of sodium for the same age group population was 2.43–5.64 for men and 1.96–3.41mg per day for women [29]. It is reasonable to assume that such an amount of potassium and sodium in the diet is adequately represented in their hair median concentration values for both men and women. In comparison, the estimated daily intake of K and Na in the white Caucasian Croatian population is considerably higher than that of the USA population [30]. However, in comparison, the US medians for a Na and K would be only lower on the common linear segment of the sigmoid saturation curve, than that for the Croatian population [15]. Thus, since the dietary intakes of K and Na are indeed represented as their hair concentration (as they are), then they would both fall well within the adequate range of their dietary intake. That leads us to the conclusion that there is no need to reduce the current level of sodium in our diet for the general population. The results urged us to provide means for the individual control of Na and K dietary intake to identify the dietary sodium overexposed subjects. Indeed, this study showed, for the first time, that there are apparently healthy subjects having a low sodium (and potassium) nutritional status. Not only their high nutritional status.

We are in no way saying that the excess dietary sodium is not harmful to the human health by inducing the increased blood pressure, especially in the salt-sensitive individuals [31], but our data indicate that there is no reason to reduce current dietary salt intake level *an block* for the general population [32, 33]. Indeed, such dietary salt reduction is a kind of "One size fit all" philosophy approach and what is certainly not justified.

With regard to the plethora of studies searching to prove the causative effect of the increased dietary salt intake on the cardiovascular system, and hypertension, in particular, we think that the respective researchers fall into the cognitive trap of the doctor Snow's water-pump handle of the cholera epidemic in London in the nineteenth century [34]. Indeed, bioelements like Na and K, when within the adequate dietary intake range, are not foreign substances to our bodies, like vibrio cholera, which is a xenobiotic bacteria; they are very much our body's essential constituents. We have discussed the issue about copying the bacteriology solutions to the trace element-specific problems in our article on assessing boron nutritional status, the time when trace element research was borrowing the concepts from the then more advanced microbiology [35].

As a matter of fact, our study does not contradict other studies where hypertension is associated with the increased urinary excretion of sodium after the increased dietary salt intake. Our study indicates that the increased urinary sodium excretion in hypertension, as observed by some researchers, is not the consequence of the increased dietary salt intake, but the failure of the cell membrane to maintain the Na and K osmotic gradient. Thus, hypertension in either the US or Croatia, is not the cause, but the effect of such an impairment. Indeed, numerous studies indicate that the impaired Na K ATPase cell membrane function may be the principal etiological cause of essential hypertension [36–39]. Our median derivatives bioassay provides a simple mean to identify the subjects at risk in the population, if and when they exceed the here proposed boundaries of the normal hair Na and K concentrations. Apparently, the essential hypertension is the "writing on the wall" that we are just aging, and that the other metabolic weakness should be also considered [40].

Acknowledgements

The initial summary of this study was partly presented at the 2015 Experimental Biology meeting (FASEB J 2015;29:S1).The author would like to thank the English language Prof. Emeritus David F. Marshall for his help with the English language.

A. Appendix

A.1 Hair potassium (H·K) and hair sodium (H·Na) analysis

A strand of hair 5–7 cm long and weighing less than one gram would be cut with titanium coated scissors over the anatomically well-defined bone prominence at the back of the skull (lat. protuberantia occipitalis externa). The individual hair samples were further minced into strands less than 1 cm long prior to chemical analysis, stirred 10 min in an ethylether/acetone (3:1, w/w), rinsed three times with the deionized H_2O (18 MΩ·cm), dried at 85°C for 1 h to constant weight, immersed one hour in 5% EDTA, rinsed again in the deionized H_2O, dried at 85°C for twelve hours, wet digested in HNO_3/H_2O_2 in a plastic tube, sonicated, and microwaved. The digested solutions were quantitatively transferred into 15 ml polypropylene test tubes. The liners and top were rinsed three times with deionized water, and the rinses were transferred into the individual test tubes. These test tubes were filled up to 15 ml with deionized water and thoroughly shaken to mix. The samples were run in NexION 300 + NWR 2013 spectrometer (Perkin Elmer, USA). Graduation of the instrument was carried out with a Perkin Elmer reference solution. We used certified GBW09101 Human Hair Reference Material (Shanghai Institute for Nuclear Research, Academia Sinica, Shanghai 201849, China, to validate the quality of the analytical work.

A.2 Whole blood potassium (WB·K) and whole blood sodium (WB·Na) analysis

Whole blood was drawn by venipuncture from v. cubiti and collected into green-cup Vacuette collecting tubes (#454082 LotA13030M7m Greineer Bio On International AG Kremsmunster, Austria) which were randomly assigned for the ICP-MS analysis. Whole blood samples of 0.5 ml were digested in a microwave oven with 0.1 ml of HNO_3 at 175° C. Blood standards were lyophilized Seronorm TM Trace Elements Whole Blood Reference Standards Level 1 (OK 0036, Level 2 (MR 9067), and Level 3 (Ok 0337) for selenium in the whole blood (SERO AS, Billingstad, Norway). Five ml of redistilled H_2O

were added to every reference standard and stirred gently at room temperature for two hours to equilibrate. One ml of such equilibrated standard was pipetted in 25 ml quartz glass vial, and dried at 105°C for 24 h. The microwaved samples were dissolved in 5 ml of redistilled H_2O with 0.1 ml of H_2O_2 added.

The detection limits for potassium (K) and sodium (Na) in the hair and whole blood were 0.0105 and 0.00105 µg·g^{-1}, respectively. All chemicals were of pro analysis grade (Khimmed Sintez, Moscow, Russia).

B. Appendix

B.1 The median derivatives bioassay (population size, PS = 1.000)

```
                                   Median (M0, µg·g-1)
<---------------------------------------------------------------->□<---------------------------------------------------------------->
Median Derivative Downward (Descending) Tail      Median Derivative Upward (Ascending) Tail
Branch (D0, PS/2 = 0.500)                        Branch (U0, PS/2 = 0.500)
Descending Median Derivatives                    Ascending Median Derivatives
D1 = D0/2        0.250                           U1 = U0 + U0/2 0.750
<-----------------------------------□------------------------------><-------------------------------□---------------------------------->
D2 = D0/4        0.125                           U2 = U1 + U0/4 0.875
<----------------□--------------->                              <----------------□---------------->
D3 = D0/8        0.062                           U3 = U2 + U0/8 0.937
<--------□------->                                                   <-------□-------->
D4 = D0/16       0.030                           U4 = U3 + U0/16        0.969
<----□---->                                                           <----□---->
D5 = D0/32       0.016                           U5 = U4 + U0/32        0.983
<□>                                                                           <□>
D6 = D0/64       0.008                           U6 = U5 + U0/64        0.992
□                                                                              □
```

We assessed the nutritional status by analyzing the frequency distribution of hair sodium and potassium and whole blood potassium and sodium with the Median derivatives bioassay. First, we assess the median (M0) hair and whole blood sodium and potassium concentration of our subject population. By definition, one-half of the studied population was above the median (upward median branch U0), and the other half was below the median (downward median branch, D0). Hence, the population size (PS) for M0 is the sum of the respective upward and downward median branches around the central inflection "hinge" M0, i.e., PS = U0 + D0 = 0.5 +0.5 = 1.0. Both the respective upward and downward median branches can be further divided in the same "median of median" way into a series of sequential median derivatives (U0,1,2,3 ... n–1, n and D0,1,2,3, ... n–1, n). For every 2 median derivative of the population, the actual hair lithium concentration can be identified. Thus, instead of mechanically throwing the preconceived percentile grid upon the observed data, we inferred the median derivative grid out from the data set itself.

C. Appendix

C.1 Potassium hair median derivatives bioassay (MDB) input data

Men (n = 339)						Women (n = 734)					
Median (M_0) = 142.5 $\mu g{\cdot}g^{-1}$ K						Median (M_0) = 73.7 $\mu g{\cdot}g^{-1}$ K					
MDB	N	K	MDC	n	K	MDB	N	K	MDC	n	K
D1	170	54.9	U1	170	486.4	d1	367	31.6	u1	367	249.5
D2	85	25.8	U2	85	1079.0	d2	184	18.8	u2	184	466.5
D3	43	16.4	U3	43	1584.0	d3	92	12.2	u3	92	857.5
D4	22	9.6	U4	22	2087.5	d4	46	8.3	u4	46	1316.0
D5	11	6.2	U5	11	3293.9	d5	23	5.7	u5	23	2629.0
D6	6	4.5	U6	6	3694.6	d6	12	4.8	u6	12	4757.9

Potassium whole blood median derivatives bioassay input data											
Men (n = 83)						Women (n = 125)					
Median (M_0) = 1369.0 $\mu g{\cdot}g^{-1}$ K						Median (M_0) = 1324.0 $\mu g{\cdot}g^{-1}$ K					
MDB	N	K	MDC	n	K	MDB	N	K	MDC	n	K
D1	42	1211.0	U1	42	1710.8	d1	63	1128.0	u1	63	1951.5
D2	21	1169.0	U2	21	2227.0	d2	32	1081.0	u2	32	2216.0
D3	11	1131.0	U3	11	2492.0	d3	16	992.0	u3	16	2286.0
D4	6	1090.5	U4	6	2702.5	d4	8	915.5	u4	8	2430.3
D5	3	1046.0	U5	3	2941.5	d5	4	558.7	u5	4	2658.5
D6	2	1021.0	U6	2	3059.3	d6	2	228.8	u6	2	6353.0

Men: Capital letters (D1 – D6, U1 – U6), Women: small letters (d1 – d6, u1 – u6).

C.2 Hair sodium median derivatives bioassay (MDB) input data

Men (n = 339)						Women (n = 734)					
Median (M_0) = 371.5 $\mu g{\cdot}g^{-1}$ Na						Median (M_0) = 254.0 $\mu g{\cdot}g^{-1}$ Na					
MDB	N	Na	MDC	n	Na	MDB	n	Na	MDC	n	Na
D1	170	146.3	U1	170	800.0	d1	367	613.3	u1	367	613.3
D2	85	84.0	U2	85	1450.0	d2	184	55.4	u2	184	1306.7
D3	43	57.1	U3	43	2035.4	d3	92	31.4	u3	92	2238.8
D4	22	34.2	U4	22	2910.5	d4	46	21.3	u4	46	3829.5
D5	11	25.1	U5	11	4015.0	d5	23	13.3	u5	23	5606.0
D6	6	12.4	U6	6	7925.0	d6	12	9.6	u6	12	7294.6

Whole blood sodium median derivatives bioassay (MDB) input data											
Men (n = 83)						Women (n = 126)					
Median (M_0) = 1780.0 μg·g^{-1} Na						Median (M_0) = 1819.0 μg·g^{-1} Na					
MDC	N	Na	MDC	n	Na	MDC	n	Na	MDC	n	Na
D1	42	1574.0	U1	42	1965.8	d1	63	1624.0	u1	63	2126.0
D2	21	1438.0	U2	21	2109.0	d2	32	1503.0	u2	32	2348.8
D3	11	1039.9	U3	11	2172.5	d3	16	1206.1	u3	16	2513.0
D4	6	895.0	U4	6	3940.1	d4	8	801.1	u4	8	6204.8
D5	3	881.8	U5	3	4805.5	d5	4	415.9	u5	4	8487.3
D6	2	564.4	U6	2	4955.0	d6	2	226.6	u6	2	10157.4

MEN: Capital letters (D1 – D6, U1 – U6), Women: small letters (d1 – d6, u1 – u6).

Author details

Berislav Momčilović
Institute for Research and Development of the Sustainable Eco Systems (IRES), Zagreb, Croatia

*Address all correspondence to: berislav.momxilovic#gmail.com

References

[1] Gaw A, Murphy MJ, Cowan RA, O'Reilly DSJ, Stewart MJ, Shepherd J. Clinical Biochemistry. Edinburgh: Churchill and Livingstone; 2004

[2] Emsley J. Nature Building Blocks. Oxford: Oxford University Press; 2003

[3] Mente A, O'Donnel MJ, Rangarajan S, McQueen MJ, Poirier P, Wiegelosz A, et al. Association of urinary sodium and potassium excretion with blood pressure. New England Journal of Medicine. 2014; **371**:601-611

[4] O'Donnel MJ, Yusuf S, Mente A, Gao P, Mann JF, Teo K, et al. Urinary sodium and potassium excretion, mortality and cardiovascular events. New England Journal of Medicine. 2014;**371**:612-623

[5] Fillipiou CD, Tsiouif CT, Thomopoluous CG, Mihas CC, Dimitriadis KS, Sotiripoulou L, et al. Dietary approaches to stop hypertension (DASH) diet and blood pressure reduction in adults with and without hypertension: A systemic review and meta analysis of randomized controlled trials. Advances in Nutrition. 2020;**11**:1-11

[6] Institute of Medicine. Dietary Reference Intakes for Water, Potassium, Sodium, Chloride and Sulfide. Washington, DC: National Academies. 2005;**11**

[7] Taube G. The (political) science of salt. Science. 1998;**281**:898-907

[8] Heaney RP. How and how not to set a nutrient intake. American Journal of Hypertension. 2013;**26**:1194-1197

[9] McCarron DA. What determines human sodium intake: Policy or physiology? American Nutrition Society. 2014;**5**:578-584

[10] Kelly JR, McGrath JE. On Time and Method. Newbury Park, CA: SAGE Publications Inc.; 1988

[11] Bankir L, Perucca J, Norsk P, Bouby N, Damgaard M. Relationship between sodium intake and water intake. Annals of Nutrition & Metabolism. 2017; **70**(Suppl. 1):51-61.

[12] Cade JE, Burley VJ, Warm DEL, Thompson RL, Margettis BM. Food frequency questionnaires : A review of their design, validation, and utilisation. Nutrition Research Reviews. 2004;**17**:5-22

[13] Xu J, Du X, Bal J, Fang L, Liu M, Ji N, et al. Assessment and validation of spot urine in estimating the 24-h urinary sodium, potassium, and odium/potassium ratio in Chinese adults. Journal of Human Hypertension. 2019. DOI: 10.1038/s41371-019-0274-z

[14] Dahm CC. Correcting measurement error in dietary exposure assessments: No piece of cake. American Journal of Clinical Nutrition. 2020;**11**

[15] Momčilović B, Prejac J, Skalny AV, Mimica N. In search of decoding the syntax in human hair. A critical overview. Journal of Trace Elements in Medicine. 2018;**45**:1-12

[16] Ehleringer JR, Avalos CA, Tipple BJ, Valenzuela VO, Cerling TE. Stable isotope in hair reveals dietary protein source with links to socioeconomic status and health. PNAS. 2020

[17] Momčilović B, Prejac J, Brundić S, Morović S, Skalny AV, Mimica N, et al. An essay on human and elements, multielement profies and depression. Translational Neuroscience. 2010;**1**: 122-134

[18] Brown M. Character of rights is adopted in the UN. New York Times. 2005

[19] Oppenheim N. Questionnaire—Design, Interviewing and Attitude Measurement. London, UK: Continuum; 1992

[20] International Atomic Energy Comission (IAEA). Elemental Analysis of Biological Materials. IAEA-TEC.DOC 197. Vienna, Austria: International Atomic Energy Agency; 1980

[21] Burges C. Valid Analytical Methods and Procedures. Cambridge, UK: The Royal Society of Chemistry; 2000

[22] Heyes B. Foolproof and Other Mathematical Meditations. Cambridge, MA: The MIT Press; 2017

[23] Finney DJ. Probit Analysis: A Statistical Treatment of the Sigmoid Response Curve. 2nd ed. Cambridge, UK; 1952

[24] Bray GA. In the footsteps of Wilbur Olin Atwater: The Atwater Lecture for 2019. Advanced Nutrition. 2020. DOI: 10.1039/advances/nmz128

[25] Schutte KH. The Biology of Trace Elements. London, UK: Croasby, Lookwood and Son. Ltd; 1964

[26] Calabrese EJ, Baldwin LA. U-shaped dose-response in biology, toxicology, and public health. Annual Review of Public Health. 2001;**22**:14-33

[27] Sanders CL. Radiation and the linear no-treshold Assumption. Heidelberg, Germany: Springer; 2010

[28] Smith SR, Klotman PE, Svetkey LP. Potassium chloride lowers blood pressure and causes natriuresis in older patients with hypertension. Journal of American Society of Nephrology. 1992;**2**: 1302-1309

[29] Institute of Medicine. Dietary Reference Intakes: Water, Potassium, Sodium, Chloride and Sulfate. Washington DC: The National Academies Press; 2004

[30] Jelaković B, Reiner Ž. Croatian Action on Salt and Health (CRASH). Zagreb, Croatia: Liječnički vjesnik; 2014. pp. 304-305

[31] Messerli FH, Schmieder RE, Weir MR. Salt. A perpetrator of hypertensive target organ disease. Archives of Internal Medicine. 1977;**157**:2449-2452

[32] Graudal N, Hubeck-Graudal T, Jurgens G, McCaron DA. The significance of duration and amount of sodium reduction intervention in normotensive and hypertensive individuals. A meta analysis. Advanced Nutrition. 2015;**6**:169-167

[33] Moore L, Singer M, Bradley ML. Low sodium intakes are not associated with lower blood pressure levels among the Framingham offspring study adults. Experimental Biology. 1917;**446**(6)

[34] Johnson BS. The Ghost Map. New York: Riverhead; 2006

[35] Prejac J, Skalny AA, Grabeklis AR, Uzun S, Mimica N, Momčilović B. Assessing the boron nutritional status by analyzing its cumulative frequency distribution in the hair and whole blood. Journal of Trace Elements in Medicine and Biology. 2018;**45**:50-56

[36] Hamlyn JM, Ringel R, Schaeffer J, Levinson PD, Hamilton BP, Kowarski AV, et al. A circulating inhibitor of (Na+ + K+) ATPase associated with essential hypertension. Nature. 1982;**300**:650-652

[37] Kramer HJ, Glanzer K, Sorger M. The role of endogenous inhibition of Na-K-ATPase in human hypertension—Sodium pump activity as a determinant of peripheral vascular resistance. Clinical and Experimental Hypertension. 1985;7: 769-782

[38] Kita S, Iwamoto T. Mechanisms for linking high salt intake to vascular tone: Role of Na(+) pump and Na+/Ca2(+) exchanger coupling. Yakugaku Zasshi. 2010;**130**:1300-1405

[39] Jailovich A, Bertorello AM. Salt, Na+, K+ -ATPase and hypertension. Life Science. 2010;**86**:73-78

[40] Miller JZ, Weinberger MH, Daugherty SA, Fineberg NS, Christian JC, Grim CE. Heterogeneity of blood pressure to dietary sodium restriction in normotensive adults. Journal of Chronic Diseases. 1987;**40**: 245-250